Current concepts in
DYSLEXIA

Current concepts in
DYSLEXIA

Edited by

JACK HARTSTEIN, B.S., M.D.

Assistant Professor of Clinical Ophthalmology, Washington University
School of Medicine; Ophthalmological Consultant to the Northwest
Educational Complemental Center of
Evaluation of Reading Disorders, Saint Louis

With 34 illustrations

THE C. V. MOSBY COMPANY

SAINT LOUIS 1971

CONTRIBUTORS

LEONARD V. BECKER, A.B., M.S.
Speech Pathologist, Audiologist, Miami, Florida

RICHARD W. BURNETT, Ph.D.
Professor of Education and Director of the Normandy UMSL Reading Clinic,
University of Missouri, St. Louis, Missouri

HARVEY EDWARD CANTOR, M.D.
Assistant Professor of Pediatrics and Neurology,
St. Louis University School of Medicine,
St. Louis, Missouri

JACK HARTSTEIN, B.S., M.D.
Assistant Professor of Clinical Ophthalmology, Washington University School of Medicine;
Ophthalmological Consultant to the Northwest Educational Complemental Center of
Evaluation of Reading Disorders, St. Louis, Missouri

JANE HURTT, Certified Orthoptist
Orthoptic Technician, Orthoptic Department, Washington University School of Medicine,
St. Louis, Missouri

MARLIN JACKOWAY, B.S., M.A., Ph.D.
Project Director, Northwest Educational Complemental Center;
Educational Counselor, Pattonville School District,
Maryland Heights, Missouri

ELEANORE T. KENNEY, Ph.D.
Director of Miriam School for Treatment of Learning Disorders, St. Louis, Missouri

MARILYN McNAMEE LAMB, B.S., M.S.
Psychological Examiner, St. Louis County Special School District; Psychologist and
Psychometrist, Department of Otolaryngology, Division of Speech Pathology, Jewish Hospital,
St. Louis, Missouri

MARK A. STEWART, M.D.
Professor of Psychiatry and Associate Professor of Pediatrics,
Washington University School of Medicine,
St. Louis, Missouri

PATRICIA TOOLEN, B.S., M.S.
Educational and Language Therapist, Department of Otolaryngology,
Division of Speech Pathology, Jewish Hospital,
St. Louis, Missouri

Dedicated to

ALL THOSE CONCERNED WITH STUDENT EDUCATION

A personal dedication to

MERLE
ANNE
MORRIS
and
LARRY

PREFACE

The term *dyslexia* holds many meanings for many people. There is tremendous interest on a national scale in this subject, which we will take to mean a condition in children with normal intelligence who have learning disorders.

The purpose of this book is to provide the reader with both an overall view of the terms, people, and studies involved in the evaluation of such children and also to provide the reader with an in-depth discussion from the points of view of the various specialists whose daily job involves them with these problems. Thus, one will gain an entire perspective of this field and be provided with the detailed thoughts of various specialists that he wishes to follow.

Unlike other books on the same subject, this book is not meant to be a team effort in which specialists complement each other so that the child is helped by a sum total of the various disciplines. In actual practice this does not prove to be the case. For example, a certain amount of controversy exists both as to the nature and definition of dyslexia and the methods of diagnosis and treatment. Reading specialists feel that these children properly fall within their province and that they should have the major, if not the entire, role. Therefore, I felt that we should expose the reader to the thoughts of the various disciplines involved so that he can gain an understanding of not only the types of disciplines that are concerned with children with learning disorders but also the approach that each one uses. The reader will soon note that certain disciplines supplement and complement each other while others steer an independent course. Through this approach the reader will not only gain an insight for himself into dyslexia but will be in a better position to counsel those of his patients who require such services.

This book came about because of my own particular interest in learning more about what to me was an unknown field. I wish to acknowledge and express my indebtedness first to Marlin Jackoway, the Project Director of the clinic with which I am associated (who originally interested me in this field), and second to the excellent and outstanding group of contributors who were kind enough and willing to join me in this undertaking. Without their help this book would not have been possible for I am certainly no expert on this subject nor do I claim to be. I am humbly grateful for the privilege of having these people join me in this venture.

JACK HARTSTEIN

CONTENTS

INTRODUCTION

The term *dyslexia* was originally introduced by Dr. Rudolph Berlin (1833-1897) of Stuttgart. He was a distinguished ophthalmologist with a strong interest in neurology and comparative ophthalmology. Since that time, the term has been variously in and out of vogue, but through most of the decades of this century has been subordinated to the descriptive phrase "word blindness." In the late fifties and early sixties, the term *dyslexia* came into high vogue and became the center of much confusion surrounding vagaries of definition. Fortunately, in the last few years the term has emerged, largely as intended by Dr. Berlin, to designate a specific difficulty in the interpretation of symbols in individuals commonly of average or above-average performance IQ. This specific, primary, or developmental dyslexia appears to have a genetic determination manifest more commonly in males than in females. In general, end organs of sensory systems such as the eyes show no gross impairment or disturbance of causal relation to the neurologic deficit.

In common with all logical processes of mankind, reasoning in regard to symbolic confusion tends to proceed from the known to the unknown. Therefore, neurologists, neurophysiologists, and neuro-anatomists have tended to fix on lesions known to be associated with *alexia*—less desirably called *acquired dyslexia*—in which a known previous ability to read has been lost. Approximately a hundred years of careful studies and postmortem documentation, predominantly in the adult, have identified causative lesions in the temporoparietal lobe or angular gyrus resulting from vascular accidents, tumors, or injuries. Uncertainty and scientific hazard, however, surround the extrapolation of such fixed adult brain pathology to the malleable child's brain. Very few brains of children with dyslexia have come to autopsy and, generally, these have not been examined in the most desirable or exhaustive detail. There is a tremendous need to study, hopefully localize, and perhaps understand something of the specific brain disturbance in children with dyslexia.

Though the hard-core problems in symbol confusion or specific dyslexia apparently represent only a small percentage of youngsters with reading retardations or learning disabilities, the uncertain alterations in neurophysiology and neuro-anatomy require much more productive understanding. Until the specific bases of disturbance are delineated, it is essential to refine functional descriptions and provisional subdivisions of clinical manifestations. In this way, the expressivity of still-undescribed lesions can be helpfully catalogued and subsequently analyzed in terms of currently available or future therapy.

Family physicians, pediatricians, neurologists, and ophthalmologists all share the obligation to deliver the healthiest possible child to the educator for the orderly progression of learning experiences. Both major and minor functional disturbances, as well as structural abnormalities, should be brought into the best possible control for the teacher. Seizures should be eliminated. Necessary glasses should be prescribed for significant symptoms. Diabetes should be controlled and thyroid function should be brought into appropriate level. None of these measures directly treat the cortical process of symbol confusion, but they may well enhance the attention span and receptiveness of the child to the learning experience. As there are no specific surgical procedures and no true learning drugs or "smart pills," the real load of treatment by educational techniques comes squarely to rest on classroom and remedial instructors. The skilled teacher quickly perceives that a child may be predominantly an auditory or predominantly a visual learner; in the presence of more severe deficit, the tactile and even the kinesthetic routes of stimulus input must be utilized. In the overall problem the therapist utilizes every appropriate route of cognitive association or sensory augmentation by the visual, auditory, tactile, and kinesthetic modalities. Simple divertissements and games also have "coffee break" value and offer a frustrated child opportunity to find some success in a world that seems symbolically stacked against him.

Thus *Current Concepts in Dyslexia* has required a multiple disciplinary approach in diagnosis but largely a unidisciplinary approach in treatment. To this end, the editor and these authors bring to bear their dedication and their individual resources in behalf of the dyslexic child. Unlike for the adult with alexia, prognosis for the dyslexic child is encouraging and is best when appropriate sensory augmentation is begun very early in the learning process. To the diligence, patience, affection, and also understanding discipline of these teachers, all parents, all patients, and all physicians are indebted.

ARTHUR H. KEENEY, M.D., D.Sc.

Ophthalmologist-in-Chief, Wills Eye Hospital and Research Institute;
Professor and Chairman, Department of Ophthalmology,
Temple University School of Medicine,
Philadelphia, Pennsylvania

chapter 1

INTRODUCTION TO LEARNING DISORDERS FOR THE OPHTHALMOLOGIST

JACK HARTSTEIN

Innumerable cases can be cited in which children with superior ability have experienced academic failure due primarily to their inability to learn to read. The impact of this failure on social and emotional well-being through the loss of status and reduced self-image results, in many cases, in serious maladjustment. In an attempt to compensate for these losses and to regain some degree of status and self-respect, the child may resort to undesirable, overly aggressive behavior or to partial or complete withdrawal. Thus the problem is compounded until he is virtually incapacitated.

In pursuit of the task and obligation of promoting the total development of children, educators have long been perplexed by their inability to cope with some kinds of learning disability which so many children with average and above-average intelligence have encountered. These problems actually come into focus more clearly in the school situation. It would seem that educators should thus be the people to take the initiative in the identification of some of the learning disabilities. However, it is important that the services of all professional people concerned with the development of children be recruited and consulted so that a coordinated effort can be made to cope more effectively with these problems. Other professional people involved with children include pediatricians, psychiatrists, psychologists, neurologists, and ophthalmologists. Since the ophthalmologist in many instances, whether willingly or unwillingly, becomes part of the team, he should become familiar with a few of the diagnostic instruments that are now available and used by educators, particularly in the perceptual areas. It certainly behooves him to become familiar with the terminology used by the educators so that he and they can literally speak the same language and understand each other for the total betterment of child care.

DIAGNOSTIC TESTS FOR LEARNING DISORDERS

Two of the better-known tests are the Illinois Test of Psycholinguistic Abilities (ITPA) by Kirk and the Marianne Frostig Developmental Test of Visual Perception. Psycholinguistic processes are the work of neurophysiological mechanisms that deal with the acquisition and usage of normal language. The three main sets of processes are *decoding, encoding,* and *association.* Decoding is the sum total of those habits required to obtain meaning from either visual or auditory linguistic stimuli; it is the ability to comprehend auditory and visual symbols, such as spoken words or pictures. Encoding is the sum total of those habits required to express oneself in words or gestures; it is the ability to put ideas into words or gestures. Association is the sum total of those habits required to manipulate linguistic symbols internally, thus relating visual or auditory symbols in a meaningful way.

Illinois Test of Psycholinguistic Abilities

In the ITPA test, nine psycholinguistic abilities are examined. They may be listed as follows:

1. *Auditory decoding* is the ability to comprehend the spoken word. It is tested by a controlled vocabulary test to which the subject is asked to answer yes or no by voice or gesture.

2. *Visual decoding* is the ability to comprehend pictures and written words. It is tested by a picture-identification technique. The subject selects from among a set of pictures the one that is most nearly identical on a meaningful basis to a previously exposed stimulus picture.

3. For *auditory-vocal association,* one uses familiar analogies. For example, "Soup is hot; therefore ice cream is ⎯⎯⎯⎯⎯⎯."

4. To test for *visual-motor* association, the subject selects from a set of pictures the one which relates in a meaningful way to a given stimulus picture.

5. *Vocal encoding* is the ability to express one's ideas in spoken words. In testing this ability, the subject is asked to describe simple objects, such as a ball or a block. A block, for example, should be described as being square, cubic, etc.

6. *Motor encoding* is the ability to express one's ideas in gestures. This ability is tested by showing the subject an object and asking him to supply the appropriate motion for manipulating it—for example, drinking from a cup or strumming a guitar.

7. *Auditory-vocal automatic ability* permits one to predict future linguistic events from past experience, without conscious effort. Tests at this level deal with the nonmeaningful use of symbols, which permits one to give conscious attention to the content of a message while the words seem to come automatically. In listening to a speech, for example, we develop an expectation for what will be said which is based on what already been said. In a test for this ability the subject must supply the last word underlined in a test statement. For example, the examiner says: "Father is opening the can. Now the can has been ⎯⎯⎯⎯⎯⎯."

8. *Auditory-vocal sequencing ability* is the skill to reproduce the sequence of auditory symbols or a sequence of symbols previously heard. In a test for this ability the subject is given a series of numbers, such as 76226243, and is asked to correctly repeat the series. This digit repetition test is dependent on auditory memory.

9. *Visual-motor sequencing ability* is the ability to reproduce a sequence of symbols previously seen. In a test for this ability the subject is required to duplicate the order of a sequence of pictures or geometric designs that are presented to him and then removed. This test is dependent on visual memory.

Of these nine psycholinguistic abilities, the two that seem most closely related to reading are the auditory-vocal sequencing ability and the visual-motor sequencing ability.

Marianne Frostig Developmental Test of Visual Perception

The second test is the Marianne Frostig Developmental Test of Visual Perception, which is commonly used in our school systems today. It consists of five parts:

1. A test of *eye-motor coordination* involves the drawing of continuous straight, curved, or angled lines between boundaries of various widths or from point to point without a guideline. It is used for both testing and training. As a training aid it helps the child to develop reading, writing, and drawing skills. It reinforces eye-hand coordination and muscle control. It teaches visual-motor coordination.

2. *Figure-ground perception* involves perception of figures as they shift in the background and perception of figures against increasingly complex grounds: Intersecting and hidden geometric forms are used in both testing and training to help the child read words in sequence—that is, he is enabled to learn the meaning of relevant clues. The ability to distinguish figure from ground is necessary for the analysis and synthesis of words, phrases, and paragraphs, without which it is impossible to learn to read.

3. A test of *constancy of shape* involves the recognition of certain geometric figures presented in a variety of sizes, shadings, textures, and positions in space, and their discrimination from similar geometric figures. Circles, squares, rectangles, elipses, and parallelograms are used. This teaches a child to recognize, for example, that 3 + 2 when written in a horizontal manner equals 5—the same as when 3 + 2 is written vertically.

4. A test of *position in space* involves the discrimination of reversals and rotations of figures presented in series. Schematic drawings representing common objects are used, for example, to teach the child to differentiate a 6 from a 9, a P from a Q, or the letter B from the letter D, as well as to discriminate between "no" and "on." In a test for this type of discrimination, a row of cats might be sitting on a fence, all with their tails turned to the right except for one cat, whose tail is turned to the left. The child is asked to indicate which one is the odd cat.

5. A test of *spatial relationships* involves the analysis of simple forms and patterns consisting of lines of various lengths and angles. The child is required to copy the lines, using dots as guide points. This test facilitates the awareness of the sequence of letters in a word. For example, after being shown a series of nine cows, in which one cow is black, the child is asked to remember which numbered cow is black.

DEFINITION OF VISUAL PERCEPTION

Before proceeding specifically to the specific role the ophthalmologist must play, let us first consider a brief definition of visual perception. There are many definitions, and they vary according to the point of view of the user of the term. One definition is that visual perception is the interpretation of sensory stimuli into the organization that leads finally to understanding, or conception. A second and perhaps more complete definition is that visual perception is the ability to recognize stimuli. This ability includes not only the reception of sensory impressions from the outside world and from one's own body but the capacity to interpret and identify the sensory impressions by correlating them with previous experiences. This process of recognition and integration of stimuli occurs in the brain, not in the receiving organ, such as the eye or the ear. For example, vision takes place in the occipital lobe, and from here the impulse passes into the angular gyrus and then goes to the frontal lobes. Therefore we have three processes in visual perception—vision, perception, and conception. Perception follows four types of stimuli: visual, auditory, kinesthetic, and tactile (abbreviated by educators as VAKT). These are the stimuli that the remedial teacher uses to improve perception.

DEVELOPMENT OF VISUAL PERCEPTION

Maximum visual-perceptual development normally occurs between the ages of 3½ and 7½ years. Unfortunately a great number of children lag in perceptual development. The child has difficulty in recognizing objects and their relationships to each other in space. The distortion and confusion with which he perceives visual symbols will make academic learning very difficult if not impossible, no matter how intelligent he is.

The cause of disability in visual perception may be pathological, as in minimal brain dysfunction, or it may be nonspecific—simply a lag in perceptual development. Sometimes a problem may be the result of an emotional disturbance sufficiently severe to cause a child to pay more attention to his inner feelings and fantasies than to the stimuli of his outer environment. Whatever the cause of the emotional disturbance, it is important to the mental health of the child that the difficulty be recognized and that remedial measures be instituted as early as possible to avoid the undesirable emotional complications that inevitably result from a failure to learn. One might ask the question, is there a correlation between visual-perceptual ability and reading achievement? and the answer would be yes. Studies have shown that there is a medium-to-high correlation between visual-perceptual ability and reading achievement at the first grade level. However, this correlation diminishes at higher levels for two reasons:

1. Children learn to master the visual-perceptual tasks by means of cognitive abilities, the development of which becomes predominant at about 7½ years of age.

2. Some children have a late spurt in perceptual growth.

DEFINITION AND EVALUATION OF LEARNING DISABILITY

To further round out the picture, let us consider a definition of learning disability and how the disability can be evaluated.

Learning disability may be defined as a condition in which a child with normal intelligence experiences severe difficulties in mastering skills in one or more basic subjects.

There are essentially three approaches in evaluating learning disability: (1) diagnostic-etiological approach, (2) diagnostic-remedial approach, and (3) task-analysis approach.

The *diagnostic-etiological approach* attempts to determine the cause of disability. The services of various medical specialists, such as neurologists, pediatricians, ophthalmologists, and psychologists, as well as other personnel, are required. Special emphasis is placed on neurophysiological and neuroanatomical disorders, such as developmental defects, infections, vascular lesions, tumors, trauma, metabolic diseases, and diseases caused by such poisons as lead, tetanus toxin, or barbiturates. In this approach the diagnosis centers on the child's developmental and medical history to establish the relationship between past factors and present status. We thus look for a physical cause for the student's inability to keep pace educationally.

The *diagnostic-remedial approach* probably is the most frequently used in the schools today. This approach deemphasizes neuroanatomical and neurophysiological factors associated with learning disability and instead establishes a profile of a number of basic educational and psychological abilities, which are then used to plan effective educational remediation. It is this approach which uses the tests we have previously discussed (the Marianne Frostig Developmental Test of Visual Perception and the Illinois Test of Psycholinguistic Abilities). From these tests the examiner constructs a profile of the child's relative strengths and weaknesses, and plans are then made to overcome the apparent learning disability.

A third method, proposed by Dr. Engelmann in 1967, is the *task-analysis approach*. If a child fails to learn a particular skill or task, the teacher's effectiveness in conceptualizing the task, in breaking down the task into teachable units, and in presenting these units is carefully examined. Thus this method focuses on the curriculum and teaching methods and on the teacher, rather than on the child's disability.

There are several criticisms of the first two methods (the diagnostic-etiological approach and the diagnostic-remedial approach). They assume that a child reads poorly because of an intrinsic personal inadequacy—that is, that the cause lies within the individual—and they focus exclusively on the child in order to discover reasons for his failure. They fail to examine important outside variables, such as curriculum, teaching methods and materials, teacher expectancy, parental expectancy, and adult acceptance. The third method, the task-analysis approach, goes to the other extreme; it evaluates the curriculum and teaching methods but does not focus on the child's disability. For example, if a child fails to learn a particular skill or task, the teacher's effectiveness in breaking down the task into teachable units and in presenting these units is carefully examined.

The answer, of course, probably lies in interrelating all three methods of evaluating a child who is not able to keep up with the other members of his class.

ROLE OF THE OPHTHALMOLOGIST

What can and must the ophthalmologist do to help those patients who may have learning disabilities? I would like to discuss, first, the general responsibilities of ophthalmologists in this field; second, the specific duties, responsibilities, and testing that falls within the province of general ophthalmological practice; and third, by means of three case studies, the role of the ophthalmologist as a member of the interdisciplinary team.

General responsibilities

The ophthalmologist is the person most often consulted. He must be fully aware of the contributions that may accrue from all the other disciplines. Since most ophthalmologists in present-day practice are not members of interdisciplinary groups dealing with dyslexia, or learning problems, it behooves the individual practitioner to familiarize himself with those groups or school systems to which his patients may be referred for more detailed evaluation. A second alternative is to familiarize himself with various specialists who have a particular interest in learning problems; one may find these specialists among the pediatricians, neurologists, psychologists, and psychiatrists. In the final analysis the current treatment of reading disorders is primarily through education by use of special remedial reading techniques. Therefore the ophthalmologist should become acquainted with educators and school authorities who are interested and involved in these problems in the particular district in which he practices.

Specific responsibilities

Specifically, and from a practical point of view, the ophthalmologist may do some or all of the following in evaluating a child with a suspected learning disorder:
1. Take a careful history and include the following questions:
    a. What grade are you in?
    b. Are you having trouble reading?
    c. Is the handwriting legible?
    d. Is there a history of mirror writing?
    e. Is there a history of reversals? (Does the child write "saw" for "was"?)
    f. Is the child a slow reader?
    g. Does the child dislike reading?
    h. Does the child come from a family of poor readers?
    i. Are there any associated speech defects?

2. A complete ophthalmological examination should, of course, be done, and it includes refraction and cycloplegia where indicated, as well as complete examination for any ocular pathology, including motility.

3. A test for visual perception should be administered. In this test, in its most elementary form, the child is presented with a series of geometric drawings, consisting of a circle, a cross, a rectangle, a diamond in a vertical position, and a diamond in a horizontal position. The first step is to present all the drawings at one time on a sheet of 9 × 12 white paper, with all the drawings in order at the top of the page. The paper is then withdrawn. The next step is to place a sheet of similar-sized white paper on a table in front of the comfortably seated child. A pencil is placed in the center of the paper, and the child is asked to pick up the pencil. The examiner notes whether the child picks up the pencil with the right hand or the left hand, and whether he picks it up with one hand and transfers it to the other. Next, the child is shown the circle and asked to "make this." He is not asked to "make a circle," because that would be giving him an auditory clue. He is allowed to make the circle wherever he desires on the sheet of paper; he is not directed to make it in any particular location. In a similar fashion he is shown the cross, the rectangle, the vertical diamond, and the horizontal diamond. Each drawing is shown to the child long enough for him to see it, perhaps 10 or 15 seconds, and then it is withdrawn.

As the drawings are being made, the examiner notes the following: (a) the direction of drawing (from left to right, or right to left); (b) the continuity of the line (continuous, or reversing direction because the patient starts at one end, goes halfway, and then goes back to the beginning and goes the other way); (c) the constancy of size of the drawings (some may be much larger or smaller than the others); and (d) the order in which the drawings are made (in the original order or scattered haphazardly over the page). From these observations, various conclusions can be drawn.

Most children with so-called normal visual perception will complete these figures in a left-to-right direction, since this is the direction of writing in our culture, and they will also complete the outside of the figures in a continuous fashion. All five figures will be drawn so that their size is in relationship one to another, and many will be drawn in the original order in which they were first perceived. Children exhibiting visual-perceptual deficits will draw from right to left, start in one direction and then reverse themselves, make one drawing much larger or smaller than the others, arrange the drawings in a haphazard fashion, or perhaps be totally unable to reproduce even the simplest of these drawings.

These drawings are referred to as the Gesell Copy Form and are also used as part of the Denver Developmental Screening Tests, devised by Dr. William K. Frankenburg and Dr. Josiah Dodds. Statistically, if a child is developing normally, he should be able to copy a circle by 3.3 years fairly well. Ninety percent of children can do so at that age. In fact, 25% can do it by 2.2 years, 50% by 2.6 years, and 75% by 2.9 years. In copying a square, 25% of children are able to do this by 4.1 years, 50% by 4.7 years, 75% by 5.5 years, and 90% by 6 years.

4. The ophthalmologist can then ask the child to draw a person. This test drawing of a person will give the doctor a good idea of the maturation of his young patient. By 6 years of age, 90% can draw a man using 6 body parts; in fact, by 4.6 years the figure is 25%, by 4.8 years it is 50%, and by 5.4 years it is 75%.

The ophthalmologist as a member of the interdisciplinary team

I have heard some ophthalmologists state that the ophthalmologist should be the captain of the team in the interdisciplinary approach to dyslexia, and I have heard other ophthalmologists state that the ophthalmologist, since he is often initially the one consulted, has major responsibilities in this field and thus should be in control of the subsequent and total investigation. It is my belief that the ophthalmologist, important as his role is, should not be in charge of the entire group. As was stated earlier, the current treatment of dyslexia, being largely a matter of special educational techniques, should be under the overall supervision and direction of the various educators and school authorities.

To clarify what I feel is the proper role of the ophthalmologist, I should like to present three detailed case studies that indicate the functions of the various disciplines and how they interrelate and work together. As a member of a fine interdisciplinary team, I have had the pleasure and privilege of working with some dyslexic children and, in some small way, of helping in the overall evaluation of these patients. Each case study will be presented in its entirety, and at the end of each report, the summary letter sent to the parents of the patient will be included. The cases are actual, and all names have been omitted with the exception of the first name of the patient.

CASE 1

READING CLINIC
STAFFING

Client: *Michael*   Date: *September 22, 1967*
                                                         Age: *6 years*
Parents: Grade: *First*
Address: Birth date: *July 31, 1961*
                                                         School:
Phone: District:

Present at staffing: *Members of interdisciplinary team*

I. BACKGROUND

   SCHOOL REFERRAL: Michael was referred because of difficulty in kindergarten.

CASE 1—cont'd

PARENT INTERVIEW: Only Mrs. _____ came for the initial interview with _____ on August 4, 1967. Although she knew the interviewer from previous school records, Mrs. _____ was very nervous. She was on the verge of tears several times as she related Mike's "problem", and she has been unable to accept Mike's limitation. Plans for his future include a college education.

CHILD INTERVIEW: Mike was interviewed by _____ on August 4, 1967. He was somewhat shy and reticent at the beginning of the interview, but relaxed as we were performing the task involved in the interview. He became more hyperactive as the interview progressed. Mike was a very chubby, angelic-looking child who appeared to be accustomed to having his own way at home.

SOCIAL HISTORY: The birth was normal. Mike walked at 1 year and talked at 7 to 8 months. The family is in the lower-middle socioeconomic scale according to Warner. The parents both graduated from high school, and both are employed full time. There are only two children in the family: Debbie, 10, and Michael.

II. EDUCATIONAL ASSESSMENT

INTELLIGENCE: The Wechsler Intelligence Scale for Children (WISC) was given February 15, 1967, by _____. It was noted that Mike was very immature. The test was given in three sessions to sustain attention.

$CA* = 5\text{-}7$ $Verbal\ IQ = 96$ $Performance\ IQ = 78$ $Full\text{-}scale\ IQ = 86$

	SCALE SCORES[†]		SCALE SCORES[†]
Information	7	Picture completion	9
Comprehension	9	Picture arrangement	8
Arithmetic	11	Block design	5
Similarities	8	Object assembly	7
Vocabulary	12	Coding	5

OTHER TESTS GIVEN: An ITPA was given in the school setting March 17, 1967, by _____. Because Mike's attention span was very short, the test was given in two sessions. Mike whispered answers he was unsure of.

	LANGUAGE AGE (years-months)
DECODING:	
Auditory	4-5
Visual	5-2
ASSOCIATION:	
Auditory-vocal	4-11
Visual-motor	4-4
ENCODING:	
Vocal	3-6
Motor	4-7
AUTOMATIC-SEQUENTIAL:	
Auditory-vocal automatic	5-9
Auditory-vocal sequential	5-11
Visual-motor sequential	5-4

Mike's greatest difficulties seemed to be in association; he was a year below his CA in both the auditory and visual association. His ability to express himself verbally was two years below his CA. Mike's complete language age is 4-11.

*Chronological age = years-months.
†Scale scores refer to section on school tests—derived from tables of norms in WISC manual, The Psychology Corp., New York, N. Y.

Continued.

CASE 1—cont'd

Marianne Frostig Developmental Test of Visual Perception was given September 14, 1967, by _____. Mike presented himself as a delightful child of 6 years. Remediation was indicated in the following areas:

      1. Eye-motor coordination
      2. Figure-ground perception

III. PHYSICAL ASSESSMENT

Biopter Vision Tests, given August 4, 1967, by _____. No problems were indicated with this instrument.

Ortho-Rater—Bausch & Lomb School Vision Tester, given August 4, 1967, by _____. This test indicated a problem area of school phoria at near.

OPHTHALMOLOGIST: Dr. _____, July 27, 1967. The eye examination showed the following:

      1. 20/20 vision in each eye
      2. No refractive error
      3. Normal muscle balance
      4. On the geometric patterns, a lack of organization and a lack of directionality, but good size constancy

Impression: I find that he has a visual-perceptual defect.

PEDIATRICIAN: Dr. _____, August 24, 1967. A physical examination shows a pleasant, somewhat overweight boy; height, 49½ inches, weight 70 pounds. He is quite cooperative with his family although he is discouraged rather easily. His gait is normal; however, on hopping on one foot he easily loses his balance. He is unable to skip. Examination of the eyes, ears, nose, and throat shows that they are essentially normal; the tonsils are moderately enlarged, but there is no evidence of disease. The blood pressure is normal; the heart and lungs show no abnormality; the abdomen shows no masses; the testes are descended; and there is no hernia. The extremities are quite normal. The tendon knee flexes are normal. The boy shows rather poor gross coordination; the first attempt at finger-to-finger touching in mid-air was done unusually laboriously and without confidence; the second try was done easily.

The patient was asked to print his name. He printed Mike from right to left, with each of the reversible letters being reversed. He could not print his last name but attempted to copy by model; he did this, omitting the "I." The boy is right-eyed, right-handed, and right-footed.

Impression: This boy is probably of normal ability, with severe difficulty in learning associated with problems of perception and space relationships. It would seem clear that he will need a good deal of encouragement and special training in this area. Mrs. _____ is very defensive about her son's problems and on the whole will attempt to infantilize him if she is not given help in understanding the nature of the problem. It was explained to her that after the first tests are done we will attempt to help Mike, but that it will be a tedious, relatively prolonged process and that he will need encouragement and support at home.

NEUROLOGIST: Dr. _____, September 1, 1967. This child fits well into the so-called "clumsy child" syndrome. This is manifest by a significant degree of right-left confusion, hyperactivity, slightly impaired motor coordination, and difficulty with visual-perceptual problems. The significance of these findings was explained to the mother. The etiology of this condition is probably based on delayed maturation of the nervous system, in an uneven fashion, affecting certain areas of performance more than others. This is probably substantiated by the difference in the verbal scale

CASE 1—cont'd

and the performance scale on the WISC. It is recommended that the school be aware of the problem and that the mother be given some reassurance and helped to realize the limitations involved in Michael's performance, and also that he most likely will improve with time. He will probably need extra help when he starts school and should have some extra help to see that he utilizes what skills he has to their maximum efficiency. This should be on a low-pressure level, but should be firm and persistent. This child probably will learn in a somewhat different fashion from the rest of his classmates, and this must be recognized by the family, the patient, and the school authorities.

IV. RECOMMENDATIONS
   1. Materials and suggestions in perceptual development to classroom teacher
   2. Careful observation by clinic specialist for possible special school district placement
   3. Parent counseling (outside agency)

LETTER TO PARENTS

Dear Mr. and Mrs. _____:

In June of this year Michael was referred to the reading clinic. On August 4, Mike came in for his initial interview, at which time I explained the complete program to you. A testing sequence was initiated, with the following results.

The clinic administered an ability test, a language test, and a visual-perception test. We found his verbal ability to be in the average range but his performance ability to be below average. His language ability was low in association from both auditory and visual stimuli. His communicative skills were below his chronological age also. His visual perception was deficient in eye-motor coordination and figure-ground perception.

Mike was seen by the ophthalmologist on July 27, the pediatrician on August 24, and the neurologist on September 1. The ophthalmologist reported 20/20 vision in each eye, with a lack of organization and directionality. This impression is that there is a visual-perceptual defect. The pediatrician believes that this is a boy of normal ability with severe difficulty in learning, associated with problems in perception and space relationships. The neurologist finds a significant degree of right-left confusion, hyperactivity, impaired motor coordination, and difficulty with visual-perceptual problems.

It is the recommendation of our reading clinic that Mike's teacher be provided with materials in visual-perception training and language development. A reading clinician will consult with the teacher weekly concerning Mike's progress and adjust materials as needed. At the end of the first semester, we will evaluate Mike's progress and will arrange another conference with you.

It is further suggested that the parents participate in a discussion group on child behavior and development.

Sincerely,

Reading Program Director

CASE 2

READING CLINIC
STAFFING

Client: *Jory*

Parents:
Address:

Phone:

Date: *August 24, 1967*
Age: *7 years*
Birth date: *November 21, 1959*
Grade: *Second*
School:
District:

Present at staffing: *Members of interdisciplinary team*

I. BACKGROUND

SCHOOL REFERRAL: Jory was referred to the reading clinic on June 15, 1967 by _____ with the following problem: Jory seems to be mentally alert but has some perceptual problems, although his coordination looks generally all right. Jory's behavior is less controlled than it was last year, and he seems to need quite a bit of attention. Academic progress has not come along, since he is finding other ways of receiving attention. The following solutions were attempted: Jory has worked in group counseling sessions and had some work on perceptual skills activities. He needs more definitive evaluation; he has made little progress despite a great deal of time and individual attention.

PARENT INTERVIEW: Mrs. _____ was present for the initial interview with _____ on June 30, 1967. The mother was attractively dressed and pleasant. She describes Jory as a thinker; she feels his ability is above average and that it is hard for him to concentrate because of this. She calls him a "vibrant" individual. Her usual reaction to him is teasing, because she feels he is unsophisticated; yet this vulnerability is what worries her most about him.

CHILD INTERVIEW: Jory was interviewed by _____ on June 30, 1967. Jory's physical appearance is somewhat deviant from the "average." His right eye goes inward when he focuses, his mouth is open for breathing most of the time, and his head is slightly pointed. He appears to have difficulty hearing. Sound substitutions were observed in his speech. He stares blandly and is difficult to communicate with. Answers to questions were bizarre. It appears that this is related to the child's inability to deal with abstraction.

SOCIAL HISTORY: Family is on the upper-middle socioeconomic level according to the Warner scale. The father has an engineering degree, and the mother has completed two years of college. They are in their thirties. There are five children in the family: Tara, 13; Dana, 11; Shaye, 9; Jory, 7; and Lauren, 4. The parents do not include their children in trips, activities, etc. During pregnancy, the mother had German measles (at 2 months). Jory walked at 12 months and talked at 18 months. He was very ill with measles at 9 months (high temperature). He was hit in the head with a baseball bat at the age of 4 years. Jory insists that his mother tuck him in bed every night. The mother states that this is the only child with this reaction. She says discipline is not a problem; however, sometimes he is very excitable and strong.

CASE 2—cont'd

II. EDUCATIONAL ASSESSMENT

DECODING:	LANGUAGE AGE (years-months)
Auditory	6-5
Visual	8-9
ASSOCIATION:	
Auditory-vocal	7-3
Visual-motor	7-6
ENCODING:	
Vocal	4-5
Motor	4-2
AUTOMATIC-SEQUENTIAL:	
Auditory-vocal automatic	7-3
Auditory-vocal sequential	4-4
Visual-motor sequential	4-10

A great deal of difficulty was displayed in giving back information that was heard and assimilated. He also seemed unable to handle auditory and visual stimuli in a sequential pattern commensurate with his overall language development (5-10).

A Frostig test was given July 31, 1967, by _____. It was noted that there was a low frustration threshold and that the work was done too rapidly and in random fashion. The left hand was used. Remediation was indicated in the following areas:

2. Figure-ground perception
3. Form constancy

III. PHYSICAL ASSESSMENT

Biopter Vision Tests were given July 3, 1967, by _____. No problems were indicated in any areas, with the exception of the acuity tests, which were invalid due to lack of knowledge of the alphabet.

OPHTHALMOLOGIST: Dr. _____, July 11, 1967. The eye examination showed the following:

1. 20/20 vision in each eye
2. No internal or external ocular pathology
3. No refractive error
4. On the geometrical pattern testing, a marked deficit, as follows:
   a. Poor directionality
   b. Confusion patterns
   c. Disorientation patterns
   d. Disorganization of the size patterns

Impression: This child definitely shows a marked visual-perceptual deficit.

PEDIATRICIAN: Dr. _____, August 10, 1967. A physical examination reveals a boy who is rather shy but not obviously fearful. His head is a little "tower"-shaped and seems slightly small. The eyes, nose, and throat are normal. There is no glandular enlargement. The heart, lungs, abdomen, genitals, and extremities are normal. The boy is moderately flat-footed. His gait is a bit awkward. His knee jerks are hyperactive, as are the ankle jerks. The Babinski reflexes are normal. There is a suggestion of ankle clonus on both sides. The boy shows dysdiadochokinesia. His speech is quite soft and seems immature. The blood pressure is normal.

Continued.

CASE 2—cont'd

The patient is right-eyed, left-handed, and left-footed. His attempt to perform a few designs of the Bender-Gestalt test strongly suggests an organic problem.

Impression: This boy has organic perceptual difficulties that impair his learning and that will necessitate special training. One cannot be sure whether the German measles in the mother was the cause of this, although it is possible. I am not sure whether mixed dominance is particularly important in this boy, although the family traits may compound his problems. It would seem useful to have a thorough neurological examination and perhaps an EEG.

NEUROLOGIST: Dr. _____, August 10, 1967.

Impressions: This 7-year-old white male has many developmental lags, behavioral and social immaturity and very obvious visual-perceptual deficits, with a fairly severe reading disability. The child is quite sensitive and aware of these limitations. The etiology is unclear—most likely it is congenital and probably familial. The disability correlates readily with the WISC score of 91, and there is no verbal and performance scale discrepancy. In general, this appears to be a dull-normal lad who is being required to perform at a level that he is incapable of accomplishing because of a deficit in visual perception, fine-motor coordination, and language development, which is additive to the above problem. I see no emotional problems nor a latent severe behavioral disorder present at this time.

Suggestions: I would agree with pediatrician that a training program designed for children with visual-perceptual problems and latent reading disorders be attempted. Its success will have to be determined by trial and error. An interpretation of the child's limitations to the parents is also in order. An attempt at finding latent talent or motor-oriented skills such as athletics (which he does not particularly enjoy) might be stressed. Placement in a local school with children of the same native abilities would be most beneficial; the competition and the expectation in regard to accomplishments would be more realistic. I see no need for medication, an electroencephalogram, further special evaluation, or language therapy at this time. I also agree with the pediatrician that this youngster's 11-year-old brother should be evaluated, either to prevent a more serious behavioral problem, or at least to make possible the aid that might come from recognizing a child with a behavioral disorder that presently exists. I would like to reevaluate this youngster after the first three months of the coming school year.

IV. RECOMMENDATIONS

The reading clinic has recommended the following:

1. Jory should be included in the regular classroom reading program, as he is only one-half grade below reading expectancy for his mental age.

2. Emphasis should be placed within the classroom program on strengthening his ability to give back information orally.

3. Auditory and visual sequencing tasks should be given within the classroom program.

4. Visual-perception training should be given by a reading clinician, three days a week for ten weeks, at which time his progress will be evaluated.

5. The parents should be assisted in arriving at more realistic goals for Jory than they now maintain.

CASE 2—cont'd

LETTER TO PARENTS

Dear Mr. and Mrs. _____:

In June of this year Jory was referred to the reading clinic by _____ school. On June 30, Jory came in for his initial appointment, at which time I explained the program to you.

A testing sequence was then initiated, with the following results: The clinic administered an ability test, a reading test, a language test, and a visual-perception test. All were individual measurements. We found his general ability to be in the average range, his reading ability to be at the middle of the first grade, and his language ability depressed in both motor and vocal communication, as well as in sequential areas. Visual perception was deficient in figure-ground perception and in recognizing constancy of form.

Jory was seen by the ophthalmologist on July 11; the pediatrician on August 10; and the neurologist on August 11. The ophthalmologist reported 20/20 vision in each eye and a marked visual-perceptual deficit. The pediatrician indicated that Jory has organic perceptual difficulties and mixed dominance. The neurologist reported developmental lags, with obvious visual-perceptual deficits, fine-motor coordination deficits, and immature language development. The neurologist would like to see Jory again in the last of November.

It is recommended by the reading clinic that Jory's teacher be provided with materials in visual-perception training and language development. A reading clinician will consult with her weekly concerning Jory's progress and adjust materials as needed. At the end of this semester, we will evaluate Jory's progress and will arrange a conference with you at that time.

Sincerely,

Reading Program Director

CASE 3

READING CLINIC
STAFFING

Client: *Richard*

Parents:
Address:

Phone:

Date: *August 28, 1967*
Age: *9 years*
Birth date: *July 3, 1958*
Grade:
School:
District:

Present at staffing: *Members of interdisciplinary team*

I. BACKGROUND

SCHOOL REFERRAL: Ricky was referred to the reading clinic on May 29, 1967,

Continued.

CASE 3—cont'd

with the following problem—he has been a nonreader. The following solution was attempted: working in the Initial Teaching Alphabet (ITA); needs continuation so that he can be back to traditional orthography in September—working in book 3, third story.

SCHOOL CUMULATIVE RECORD: Iowa Tests of Basic Skills, given in the school, gave the following pertinent scores:

October, 1966, Subtest		*April, 1967, Subtest*	
GE*	PR†	GE*	PR†
Vocabulary: 18	Vocabulary: 12	Vocabulary: 21	Vocabulary: 9
Reading: 25	Reading: 31	Reading: 19	Reading: 4

During the second grade no grades were given and the parents were advised by conference and letter of Ricky's progress. Despite poor grades and inability to do the work, Ricky has never been retained until this year; and this was only at the parents' request.

PARENT INTERVIEW: Mrs. _____ was present for the initial interview with _____ on June 21, 1967. The mother was very talkative. She is very interested in obtaining help for Ricky and will be glad to have him in the program. She does not, however, want Ricky to have another EEG, as she feels that the experience is too traumatic. Mrs. _____ feels that all of Ricky's coordination problems are probably due to a severe burn, although she says many doctors have told her that this is not so. She is also concerned about how and when to explain his adoption to Ricky.

CHILD INTERVIEW: Ricky was interviewed by _____ on June 21, 1967. He appeared as a pale, average-sized, 8-year-old. He was extremely active during the interview, and communication was difficult. At times he would stare into space and was, for a moment, not involved in his immediate environment. It was necessary on several occasions to bring him back verbally or by touching him. He appeared immature and overly dependent on his mother. The interviewer asked him if he would like to remove his jacket, and Ricky turned to his mother for approval.

SOCIAL HISTORY: The family is on the upper-middle socioeconomic level according to the Warner scale. Ricky was adopted at 5½ months of age. The mother's pregnancy and birth were normal as far as adoption. At 10½ months Ricky was severely burned. He was in his walker and pulled the cord of the coffeepot, spilling the coffee on his neck and back. Ricky is an only child, and Mr. and Mrs. _____ take him many places with them.

OTHER AGENCIES: Report from _____, Inc., dated May 4, 1966. The testing indicates that Ricky is a boy of above-average intellectual capacity who gradually needs to learn by making his own mistakes and gradually needs more independence at home. He needs to learn to assert himself, by himself, and to make small mistakes by himself at the same time that he is protected from larger ones. In addition, he needs to improve his approach to reading, writing, vocabulary, and study. His comprehension, recognition of similarities, and understanding of content are excellent. It is in the skill areas that he needs to be brought up to something approaching more closely his level of ability. Basically, although he has some mild anxiety, he is a normal child and now needs to accelerate his emotional and social development, which in turn will free him and help him, as soon as he masters the reading, to accelerate tremendously his academic achievement.

*Grade equivalent.
†Percentile rank.

CASE 3—cont'd

II. EDUCATIONAL ASSESSMENT

INTELLIGENCE: The Wechsler Intelligence Scale for Children was given August 15, 1967. It was noted that Ricky seemed to wander on vocabulary words and did not seem to want to try. He would not give answers but could use the words correctly in sentences later in the test. In all areas, it was necessary to obtain absolute attention before proceeding with the test.

$CA* = 9\text{-}1$ $MA* = 0\text{-}11$ Verbal $IQ = 89$ Performance $IQ = 115$ Full-scale $IQ = 101$

	SCALE SCORES		SCALE SCORES
Information	9	Picture completion	12
Comprehension	7	Picture arrangement	14
Arithmetic	11	Block design	10
Similarities	13	Object assembly	14
Vocabulary	1	Coding	11

The *Stanford-Binet* vocabulary test was given August, 1967. Ricky passed the year X level.

The *Bender Visual-Motor Gestalt for Young Children* was given August, 1967, and indicated no severe perceptual problem or emotional lability.

READING: The Spache *Diagnostic Reading Scales* were given July, 1967. Ricky appeared immature for his age, with some baby talk. He required constant reassurance. The following things were noted: (1) reversals, both letter and word; (2) substitution of nonrelated words; (3) addition of letters to words; (4) fairly good use of consonants but limited use of vowel sounds; (5) ability to blend well when vowel sounds are known and need to point to words to keep place.

GRADE EQUIVALENT

Word recognition	2.0
Instructional level (oral)	1.8
Reading expectancy	4.03 *(MA = 9-11)*
Potential level (listening)	3.3

OTHER TESTS GIVEN: An *ITPA* was given July 24, 1967. Ricky was very cooperative during the testing; however, his speech made him hard to understand. His attention wandered frequently and he commented on previous events and pictures continuously. He has a large vocabulary and background of experiences. Language scores are as follows:

	LANGUAGE AGE (years-months)
DECODING:	
Auditory	8-10+
Visual	8-9+
ASSOCIATION:	
Auditory-vocal	7-8+
Visual-motor	8-11+
AUTOMATIC-SEQUENTIAL:	
Auditory-vocal sequential	8-6+
Visual-motor sequential	4-11

*Chronological age and mental age = years-months.

Continued.

CASE 3—cont'd

This child seems to have difficulty in relating information back when he is restricted to a single subject. He also had difficulty in sequencing designs visually.

The *Marianne Frostig Developmental Test of Visual Perception* was given on July 18, 1967. It was noted that Ricky was unsure of which hand to use and finally chose the left hand, which he used consistently throughout the test. He required constant reassurance that he was responding correctly. Remediation was indicated in the following areas:

1. Eye-motor coordination
2. Figure-ground perception
5. Spatial relations

III. PHYSICAL ASSESSMENT

Biopter Vision Tests, given July 20, 1967. A deficit in acuity on the far point test and an overconvergence in lateral phobia on the near point test were indicated.

OPHTHALMOLOGIST: Dr. _____, August 11, 1967. The eye examination showed the following:

1. Normal vision, 20/20 in each eye
2. No ocular pathology
3. Distortion in size patterns and confusion in direction, shown by perceptual form testing

Impression: A visual-perceptual problem exists.

PEDIATRICIAN: Dr. _____, August 4, 1967. A physical examination reveals a boy of 86 pounds, 54½ inches tall. He is somewhat overweight. He is at present cooperative during the examinations. His speech is somewhat immature, with some lisping. The gait is quite normal. The general physical examination shows no obvious abnormalities. The eyes, ears, nose, and throat are quite normal. The heart and lungs are clear; the abdomen is negative; the genitals and extremities are quite normal. The tendon reflexes are perhaps a little more active than normal.

Ricky's writing is extremely labored. There are excessive movements of the left hand while he is writing with the right hand. A few tests of the Bender series suggest, perhaps, some element of organicity. No mixed dominance was shown by my rough testing at this time.

Impression: It is my feeling that Ricky probably has a specific language disability, perhaps related to some mild organicity despite the negative EEG. The history of two days of shock after a burn, plus the presence of the soft signs of a hyperactive knee jerk, might be evidence to confirm this impression. It is possible that the mother is somewhat overprotective, and this might aggravate the boy's problems, but I would suspect that it is not primary. There is no indication here for drug therapy in my opinion.

NEUROLOGIST: Dr. _____, August 11, 1967. Examination disclosed Richard's mannerisms to be somewhat infantile and his speech to be somewhat impoverished. During the mental status examination, he was unable to give the date, could not repeat four digits backward, and could not name the month. He was able to make up sentences when given three specific words. He could count backward from 20 to zero. He was not able to write a four-word sentence within one minute. When he was asked some commonsense questions, his answers were somewhat impaired and probably not on the level that one would anticipate from a 9-year-old child. His performances in drawing a man and drawing a house were below that which one anticipates. His ability to write short sentences from dictation was markedly impaired. There were omission of words and incorrect spelling; how-

CASE 3—cont'd

ever, when asked to spell the words individually, for the most part he was able to do so. He was able to copy sentences without too much difficulty. His copying of geometric forms was fairly normal. He was able to follow three- or four-step commands but showed significant right-left confusion. He appears to be right-eyed, right-handed, and right-footed. The neurological examination showed that his cranial nerves are normal, his visual fields and fundi are normal, his hearing and auditory discrimination appear to be normal, and his muscle tone and strength are normal. There was a slight increase in his knee jerks, but the rest of his reflex examination was normal. His motor coordination of small movements appeared to be somewhat poorer. There was significantly more associated movement than would be normal for his age. His sensory examination within the limits of cooperation was grossly normal. His gait was normal; however, he was unable to skip.

Impression: I feel that Richard's native intellectual endowment is probably on the low side of normal. He manifests significant maturational delay in the development of his nervous system and function. This is manifested by his speech, his behavior and postures during testing, and his verbally presented material. His performance of visual-motor skills was greater than auditory-motor skills to date, although both are somewhat impaired. I would recommend repeated intelligence testing and special instruction for this youngster in the field of reading and fine motor coordination.

IV. RECOMMENDATIONS

The reading clinic has recommended the following:

1. Group reading instruction should be provided within the school remedial reading program, beginning on a first grade primer level (to build confidence) and proceeding, when ready, to the first reader. Ricky's knowledge of phonics should be used and broadened so that he can utilize it in word analysis.

2. Visual perception training should be given by a reading clinician, three days a week for a period of ten weeks, at which time his progress will be evaluated.

3. If necessary, materials and suggestions can be provided to the classroom teacher for individual seatwork activities.

4. Activities should be given to enhance Ricky's self-concept and independence. Suggestions for appropriate activities will be made to the parents and teacher by a reading clinician.

LETTER TO PARENTS

Dear Mr. and Mrs. _____:

Ricky has been given specialized reading instruction at the clinic for one hour, three days a week, for approximately one and one-half months. This instruction was based on the following diagnosis by the staff.

Normal intelligence (WISC) was found, with a reading potential of fourth grade. The Spache Diagnostic Reading Scale, however, indicates an oral reading level of high first grade and a comprehension level of about low third grade. The Marianne Frostig Developmental Test of Visual Perception indicated remediation in

Continued.

chapter 2

INTERDISCIPLINARY APPROACH TO THE DIAGNOSIS OF READING PROBLEMS

MARLIN JACKOWAY

This chapter will be devoted to the consideration of reading problems in the regular schools from the frame of reference of an educator not specializing in reading and not concerned with "special" education. I have served as the project director for a supplementary education center for a regular school district during the years 1966 to 1970. Prior to that I worked as a teacher and counselor in the regular schools. One of the major programs under my direction as project director was a reading clinic, and the views expressed below are the result of my experiences as the administrator for that section. For some time before my involvement in the supplementary center, I was interested in the problem of reading in the schools, agreeing with those who call reading disability the "leukemia" of education.

Since reading problems first become visible in the regular school, I believe that the view of a regular-school educator should be helpful to concerned professionals from other disciplines. I am not claiming the only realistic view of the problem. Rather, I will try to speak here for a group who are intimately involved in the problem from the point of recognition and who continue to live with it daily, whereas others often are less involved.

I see the problem of reading disability against the background of an advanced technological society that has a "hang-up" where reading is concerned. Children are threatened with a limited future if they do not learn to read with a certain proficiency. This is done indirectly by requiring certain levels of education for jobs that in reality require very little reading for successful performance after the applicant is hired. It is assumed that completion of a particular grade in school indicates a certain proficiency in reading—the major means of communication in the schools. This has not been the case in recent years and is a cause of confusion among both educators and the community-at-large.

As an educator, I have known children in school who, I would expect, could succeed in many vocations that do not require a great amount of reading but are unable to stay in school long enough to receive the diploma that is required for job entry, whereas others, who stay in school, are quite limited in their capacity to perform the same job. Many children with this type of problem are classified as disabled readers.

After more than ten years of observing the problems of these schoolchildren, I have become somewhat skeptical about solutions. I have seen the children attended by a multitude of specialists from many disciplines, with little help. Before the interdisciplinary approach to the diagnosis of reading problems is discussed, I believe I should share my view of the crazy-quilt pattern of approaches in the schools.

When a child is first found to be having troubles with reading, he is generally in a "regular" public-school classroom, where a multitude of programs and levels of instruction are found. The first attempts to help him will be made here, and if they fail, additional help may be offered by a reading specialist employed by the school. Such specialists may work either with small groups or individually with each child, depending on the local educational unit's capacity and willingness to offer these services.

The course open to the school becomes unclear if these efforts seem to be unsuccessful. In some cases the parents become dissatisfied with the school's efforts and seek other help, often from outside the field of education. The reasons given for seeking outside help may be the prestige of the other fields, such as medicine, the parental feeling that the educators have failed, the unwillingness of the schools to make outside referrals, or assorted other reasons.

In some cases it seems logical to parents that their child must have a vision problem, and therefore they will seek the help of either an ophthalmologist or an optometrist. It seems to me that here they will probably meet with two different frames of reference. The medical doctor will probably find nothing wrong or possibly a slight refractive error, and will say that the reading problem is not related to vision, whereas the optometrist will be more likely to discover a vision problem and will refer the child to a colleague or embark on a program to correct the problem himself. Meanwhile, back at the school, little progress is noted in the area of reading.

Some parents may share their problem with their family physician or pediatrician. His recommendations may take various forms, depending on his orientation. He may feel that the child will probably outgrow the problem, or he may refer the child to such sources as a psychologist, psychiatrists, family and child social work agencies, neurologist, and speech correction therapist. Even when medication is involved, it is more often the case that the doctor will fail to contact the school. The educator is still left out of this type of program in most cases and continues to handle the child with little knowledge of what is happening elsewhere. In some cases when the teacher is consulted, little information is shared with him. As an illustration, one social worker once told me that he did not think it wise that we discuss the case because the client might get the idea that we were "ganging up" on him. The result is that the school institutes a hands-off policy and seeks only to contain the child or to go on doing what it usually does, although that course of action may be antagonistic to the efforts of the outside agency or professional.

When the school is located near a university-operated program, or has a clinical capacity of its own or one that is available through a special agency, various other possibilities exist. For example, the program may be under the direction of educational practitioners, or it may be attached to a university school of education, medicine, or psychology, or to various combinations of schools. The program I direct had its beginning under Title III of the Elementary and Secondary Education Act of 1965 and was directed by the regular school district awarded the grant. Title III programs, like mine, usually try to bring together specialists from many different fields into an interdisciplinary group, so that the problems can be approached from as many frames of reference as possible.

It is important to point out that in some areas, where funding has been difficult or the demand for service has been very great, private groups have joined together either formally or informally to meet the needs. One of the problems with such a group, as with public groups, is that the most dominant member usually gives the program its direction, so that the cases are usually approached from one frame of reference. It seems to me that this can easily happen when the social work model of case conferences is employed—I refer to the practice in which the staff confers around a table to decide how to approach the treatment of the problem. Thus, because of the pressure of time, a multidisciplinary group performs as if there were only one discipline involved. Its movement toward an interdisciplinary operation may be very slow or nonexistent. In the same way that a one-to-one teaching situation does not guarantee individual instruction, a case conference does not always guarantee interdisciplinary functioning.

When a group defines the roles of the participating professionals and encourages interaction, there seems to be a greater chance of success. The interdisciplinary clinic seems to me, therefore, to offer the best organizational design in the face of learning problems, primarily because these problems seem to resist solution by any single discipline; by their nature, they seem to cut across disciplines. The important concept is that the team members must learn to work through the educator. Because of his position in the school, he is in a position to carry out the recommendations with the greatest saving of time and effort. He knows what the school can do and, given the benefit of what the other disciplines feel the child needs, is in the best position to weld the school's capacity to help and the recommendations of the professionals into an operational program.

THE EDUCATIONAL SETTING

When I speak of the schools, I want to make it clear that I do not believe that the schools are all the same or that all educators use the same frame of reference when considering reading problems. Programs in the regular schools range from no help at all for classroom teachers, who might have had only one or possibly two courses in reading instruction, to a comprehensive classroom program under a trained teacher who has specialized in reading and who is supported by reading teachers. Additional help may be available through a "special" education program that includes separate classrooms or itinerant teachers, or both. These extremes of program offerings may exist in neighboring school districts.

It may not be clear to some readers unfamiliar with the organization of the schools that when I speak of "regular" schools I refer to the schools most people think of when schools are mentioned. The "special" schools are for children who deviate markedly from the regular school population on at least one significant variable—hearing, seeing, mental ability, or some less well defined areas given consideration in recent years. The teachers in the special schools usually have received training that prepared them for working with a particular type of disabled child. In some colleges these programs are offered in the form of courses to be completed after regular school certification courses have been accomplished, whereas in other colleges the special educators take a different course load from that of regular teachers and arrive at the certification level without very much contact with teachers in the regular schools. This separate training often contributes to the formation of different frames of reference between special and regular educators.

Since difficulty in reading is a crippling disability for children in the regular schools, there has been a movement to consider reading as an area in which special educators should function. The category of handicapped children has been redefined to include children with reading problems as well as those classified as hard-of-seeing, hard-of-hearing, mentally retarded, orthopedically handicapped, and emotionally disturbed. Parkinson's law has been operating to some extent in this expansion, and although some regular educators have welcomed the expansion of the special programs because they offer a place to "dump" unsuccessful students, others welcome it because it offers additional revenue sources by providing services without using the local unit's tax dollar. However, the children's best interests do not seem to be served, in the opinion of most regular educators.

Children assigned to full-time special schools learn that they must have special treatment and often follow courses that lead to a dependent future, where the costs to the community must be calculated in lifetime welfare expenditures. Where a child is assigned to an itinerant teacher from a special education program, the regular-school teacher feels that his skills are limited in handling the child and therefore provides a containment environment, depending on the special teacher to correct the child's disability before demanding academic performance from him. The net result, as I see it, is an inferior educational opportunity for the child. This situation is often accompanied by a negative self-image that defeats the motivational efforts that are the key to success.

In most places the children who are placed in special classes or schools are placed there only after comprehensive evaluations conducted by qualified examiners representing various specialties, and they possess significant deviations from the average children in the regular classrooms. The frequent criticisms of special programs based on the assumption of inappropriate assignment through indiscriminate placement are just not true in my experience. What I question is the assignment to special programs of children with problems that are common enough so that programs could be maintained in the regular schools for them. I feel that children of all types benefit from comprehensive education programs if the schools are flexible enough to meet their individual needs.

One last school program, which is available to a lesser degree than the others mentioned above but still found often enough to mention, is the special clinical type of program operated by the schools themselves, in cooperation with university training programs, or by universities that accept referrals from schools. The first type of program is a supplementary program such as the one that I have directed. This program was funded under Title III of the Elementary and Secondary Education Act of 1965. Others operate through local funding, and still others have been supported by various other grants from the state or federal government and private foundations. These groups generally bring together specialists from many fields to view the children referred to the program and, depending on the model used, offer diagnosis and in some cases remediation programs.

The cooperative ventures between universities and local school districts have been found near university centers for many years. The Montreal Learning Center, the Reading Clinic at the University of Missouri at Columbia, and the Normandy Reading Clinic at the University of Missouri at St. Louis are all examples of these programs. The staffing of these programs depends very much on the frame of reference of the sponsoring group, the availability of interested specialists from other fields, and the model used.

Finally, university units that operate independently of the local schools but accept referrals from the schools are largely found at private or parochial, rather than state, universities. These units, because of administrative problems, usually function at maximum loads in after-school programs during the year and especially during the summer school terms.

During the past few years, many children living in deprived areas have been offered free summer programs in remedial and developmental reading. These programs are operated by local schools and are funded under Title I of the Elementary and Secondary Education Act. Although many children have participated in these programs, their long-term value has lately been questioned.

With all the above programs serving the schools, in some areas there still remain a hard core of children who do not learn to read at an acceptable level of proficiency. It is therefore to be expected that their parents will seek help from other sources and from specialists other than educators.

OTHER SPECIALTIES
Vision testing

Since sight seems logically to be the major sense associated with reading, most parents and many educators feel that if a child is experiencing difficulty with reading, the first place to start is with vision testing. Most schools provide routine vision screening every other year. Testing is administered by the school nurse, using a Snellen chart. Children with possible problems are identified, and parents are notified for referrals to vision specialists, usually outside the schools. Sometimes when a child is deemed to be in need and his parents have limited means, the school social worker will see that arrangements for refraction are made with a county agency or with a private organization interested in these problems. If a child is referred to a clinic type of program, his vision will probably be tested by special equipment such as the Ortho-Rater or other vision screening equipment by which visual distortions are more readily identified. In addition, tests that detect visual-perceptual difficulties, such as The Bender Visual Motor Gestalt Test for Young Children, the Beery Developmental Test of Visual-Motor Integration, or the Marianne Frostig Developmental Test of Visual Perception, are administered.

Children who fail this testing are usually referred to specialists for a more comprehensive visual examination. The practice in most schools is to have the parents check with their family physician, clinic, or optometrist. The frame of reference of the referral specialist usually predicts his recommendation to the patient. If the child does not need glasses or is on the borderline and has been referred to an ophthalmologist, the educator usually expects that the parents will be told that the child does not have a vision problem and that his reading problem is not the result of a vision problem. He may suggest a follow-up schedule to watch the problem. If an optometrist is consulted, it seems to me that the child will be more likely to receive glasses and possibly be referred for visual-perception training either by the optometrist himself or with a colleague who specializes in that type of work. A few medical doctors have been referring such children to to optometrists for programs of visual-perception training. In most cases both the ophthalmologists and the optometrists who recommend such programs are careful to make no claims for the programs beyond the correction of the visual distortion, but the implied idea is that this correction will affect the child's reading and other schoolwork. It has not been my experience that this is true at any regular or predictable rate. While the child is receiving this training outside the school, the program at the school usually follows its regular course. In some instances the specialists do communicate with the school, but this is not the rule; when they communicate, they experience a mixed reception from the school authorities.

Child psychology

A second specialist to work on the problem, often by referral from the school counselor, teacher, parents, or family physician, is the psychologist. Some psychologists have regular courses in which they work with disabled readers in groups and individually. Their frame of reference usually leads them to see the problem as one centered in the psyche rather than in the soma, although they may use pacers, tachistoscopic machines, and other equipment along with psychological techniques to attack the problem. Although there are successes with both this and the optometric therapy, there does not seem to me, as an educator, to be a sufficiently high rate of predictability in either method for the school to make referrals to the programs as they would to a medical doctor for medical help for a child. Furthermore, not all psychologists are interested in learning problems or have programs available for referral, so that the school is forced to consider individual professionals before making a referral.

Hearing testing

A third specialty that fits into the same category as vision testing and remediation is the hearing specialty. In most clinics hearing as well as vision is routinely tested, and the regular schools often have a biannual hearing testing program.

If a child fails these tests, which are usually conducted by trained audiologists using small audiometers, he is referred to his family doctor or to one of the agencies that carry on hearing testing programs. If he reaches the clinic of the regular school or of a university, he will be given another audiometer screening test under less rushed conditions than the biannual testing program allows, as well as Wepman's Auditory Discrimination Test. If he fails these tests, he will be referred for a complete work-up at a hearing agency or by a hearing specialist. Should hearing turn out to be significantly impaired, the child may be assigned to a special program and may be referred to an agency or private physician for therapy or instrument prescription.

Speech instruction

A kindred problem that affects reading is the problem of speech impairment. Children with speech difficulties are referred to speech teachers, who usually work on itinerant schedules in the regular schools from assignments in the special schools. Therapy is available to most children in the schools. However, it is often limited to one hour per week or less, and for that reason progress is often quite slow. Some parents take their children to private or public agencies with the hope of speeding up the process. The actual direct effect of this type of instruction on reading has yet to be proved to most regular educators.

Neurology

Probably the most controversial specialty involved in the problem of reading is neurology. Although it is the most controversial, I believe that my experience indicates that it is this quarter which offers the greatest hope. At present much has been written by interested neurologists about learning problems, and even more has been written by nonneurologists about what they believe the neurologists are saying. I, for one, believe that the neurologist is not ready to make any statements other than descriptive ones about the problems in reading. These specialists operate clinics and offices in children's hospitals and daily see many children with learning problems. Their most important function is to discover for the educator and the parent the true nature of the child's problem. They see the disability as developmental in nature and generally recommend that the school find ways to bypass the problem area, because they feel that the child will progress at a certain rate regardless of the school's efforts and will possibly improve at a faster rate if left alone. Here I see the psychologist and the neurologist agreeing on the handling of the problem but for different reasons. If one considers the position in which I see most of the ophthalmologists also, he may surmise that I see most medical advice as a "hands off" type of recommendation. Although this is not true on an an individual basis, it certainly is true enough as a general statement.

I do not believe that these specialists are against studying the problem, but they resist the application of techniques for the correction of reading which have not been fully investigated and proved satisfactory. This gives some educators the impression that neurologists and psychologists do not want educators to "try" with these children. Actually, the difference lies in the diagnosis of the problem. If the child has fallen behind because of poor instruction or lack of instruction, there is no question about the advantage of remedial and developmental reading instruction. However, when the instruction has been maximal and the child is still experiencing difficulty, a difference of opinion comes into the picture. The problem, then, is discovering the real reason for the child's inability to learn to read.

Not all specialists in reading education or all neurologists agree on how actual reading instruction should be given. The effectiveness of any type of drill for reading instruction as opposed to the effectiveness of allowing the child to follow his own methods has been questioned. In our program I have witnessed the modification of views held by medical, psychological, and education specialists as they came into daily contact with the specific problems of disabled readers.

INTERDISCIPLINARY GROUPS FUNCTIONING OUTSIDE THE SCHOOLS

It seems wise to continue with a discussion of the various groupings of specialties that have come into existence because of the limited funds of the schools and the growing concern of the community in this area. Since the schools have had limited monies to carry out research, and since, when the monies have been made available, the studies have been restricted to inadequate periods of time and loosely structured designs that did not permit the control of variables, little has been learned conclusively about the process of reading. This has left most of the work in the field to interested persons who operate from theories that are unproved but who seem to offer the only hope for many disabled readers.

In some cases groups of interested professionals have found the limited capacities of public programs too restrictive, and parents have increased the demand for service to such a point that the professionals have banded together in informal groups for the purpose of making referrals to each other, or in formal groups operating from shared offices during hours other than those of the public program in which the individuals are employed. These groups may be operated as nonprofit or profit associations. They usually function outside the schools but are staffed by qualified professionals and will usually function with one frame of reference.

In addition to these quasi-public and private groups of professionals, many commercial companies with special techniques or instrumentation offer to handle reading problems. Most of them are not looking for the disabled reader but prefer to work with people wishing to improve their reading speed. However, they will not turn away disabled readers and must therefore be considered as a part of the panorama that greets the regular-school educator as he views the reading scene.

It is important to point out that regular-school educators have made use of each of these methods, either for themselves or for their own children, at one time or another during the past few years. Playback from persons using these various services has been mixed, ranging from extremely successful to very negative experiences. It has therefore been my position that I will acquaint a concerned parent with the community resources but will not recommend a specific program.

Commercial programs have reached the point that one public school system, in Texarkana, contracted with a company to teach the children to read. The contract was based on a performance pay schedule, with no payment made if no improvement took place. The contract was the first of its kind and generated great interest until it was charged that the company was teaching the test. The idea is not dead, but the attitude toward it has cooled considerably, and a wise, proceed-with-caution attitude seems to prevail.

Still another group should be considered—the hospital dyslexia clinic or learning disabilities group functioning under medical direction for a limited number of clients, usually with remediation taking place at the hospital facilities under the direction of therapists using a combination of programs and techniques in clinical approaches to the problems. Being outside the schools, these clinics usually work with children in programs that are supplementary to the school rather than operating a private school.

Finally, the educator sees another group of persons operating in this area. These persons are much more difficult to describe because there is such a large range of expertise among them and because there is no regulation by any agency. These are the tutors who serve the community. They range from retired teachers to college students, and from traditionally trained reading teachers to persons without any background except that they can read.

Costs range from a few dollars an hour to "packages" amounting to $1,500, and I suspect even more, although I have not had experience with nor been told of costs in excess of $1,500. I have seen mothers go to work to support such a program for their children. The risks seem to be accepted easily, no doubt because the consequences of reading disability are so great.

INTERDISCIPLINARY GROUPS IN THE EDUCATIONAL SETTING

The integration of the school programs with the specialties mentioned above seems to me to offer the greatest hope for an emerging solution to the problem of reading disability. The ultimate program must incorporate those elements developed outside of education into the educational effort, mainly through the training of educators to employ them in their daily work. This can be accomplished only as interdisciplinary groups develop the necessary skills within the educational setting. The ultimate goal would not be the adjustment of the child but rather the rebuilding of the school program around the nature of the child as it is illuminated by interdisciplinary examination. The program would then be tailored to use the assets of the child and, where possible, to bypass his deficits.

Oakland describes the history of the diagnostic movement in survey form for those interested, and I feel that a close-up view of a particular program will be productive. I will therefore attempt to describe one inter-disciplinary unit, although I do not want to give the impression that I feel we have perfected the final form or that we have achieved complete interdisciplinary cooperation at this point.

The project I would like to describe here came into existence under the Elementary and Secondary Education Act and was part of the supplementary educational centers program. This particular center operated four other programs, but the heart of the project was the diagnostic clinic programs in guidance and reading. The center was to complement the regular-school programs. I again mention the term "regular" school because I want to make it clear that it was considered essential that the center function as an integral part of the regular-school program and not as a "special" education program or classroom.

Staff specialists

It is important to first consider the staffing of the center, because it helps explain the recommendations of the clinic and the frame of reference of the group. The full-time staff of the reading clinic included four reading specialists. All were certificated classroom teachers with special certification in reading, and one had special certification in guidance, counseling, and psychological examination. The first group that functioned during the first year was composed of persons who were selected for their diverse backgrounds and training rather than for traditional reading training. This was important because the "regular" reading teachers in the grant area were trained in traditional approaches to reading problems.

The specialists were supported by a comprehensive team of consultants. Ophthalmologists located near the center saw children who failed the vision testing on the Snellen and Ortho-Rater examinations. Almost all the children were given pediatric examinations. During the first year a comprehensive examination was employed, but during the second and third years this procedure was streamlined to a brief screening examination conducted by a team of physicians. After the pediatric screening, children were referred to a team of pediatric neurologists and to the psychiatrist as recommended. As a rule the psychiatrist would request that the psychologist see the children for projective testing prior to his examination.

In addition to the medical and psychological complement, consultants from the fields of social work and reading took an active role. First, each consultant would examine some of the children on his own and then make recommendations to the various reading specialists (educators) working with those children. Second, each consultant would review some cases that he had not seen, and then, indicating his frame of reference, make recommendations with the appropriate educators. This procedure was very difficult for the consultants and was used at a lesser rate than the personal examination method. Final write-ups, including recommendations, were monitored by each discipline to ensure proper interpretation of its recommendations, and by the director for articulation of the recommendations in the final report.

The clients of the center came from four public school districts and one parochial school district serving approximately 40,000 Midwestern suburban children. The families ranged from the lower to the upper-middle class on the Warner scale of socioeconomic status.

The clinicians of the center not only had the task of developing a format and program that would allow the various disciplines to work together but also had to consider the problems caused by serving five separate school systems. I will try briefly to describe these problems because they undoubtedly will be repeated in most communities.

First, the fear educators have of bringing medical and psychological personnel into the school stems in part from the high prestige enjoyed by these fields. Educators find themselves often overwhelmed by these consultants, who, they claim, "hit and run"—that is, they make recommendations which the educator believes are impossible to implement and then say, "See, you didn't do what I recommend—therefore, you failed." The need is for consultants with a greater knowledge of what is possible at the classroom level and with the ability to make suggestions that can be implemented in that framework.

Second, the social work/psychiatric case conference model in which the children are first viewed by all the specialists and then discussed by the group often places the ball in the hands of the most dominant member of the team. It also forces the selection of consultants from those who are free at the time of the all-important conference. These two elements, plus the time-consuming conference, are costly in terms of time and effort, and the resulting recommendations from the group generally still reflect the biases of the dominant member.

By carefully selecting the consultants, our program developed a procedure that allows both the consultant and the educator to learn more and conserve time as well. By placing in the educator's hands the responsibility to develop the diagnosis and treatment program, with constant review by consultants, we have produced a group of uniquely trained educators who understand the contributions of the various fields assisting in the program. I feel that a new respect has developed among the practitioners in the fields of education, medicine, and psychology in this setting.

Third, the elements external to the group but of significance to the client and the project include the various district programs; the vital interest in reading disability by community groups; and faculty variations in training, experience, and bias. I will attempt to explain each of these elements briefly and to discuss their implications for the project.

The various district programs, in the case of our project, include four independent public school districts and one group of parochial schools served by the project. Each school district had followed different reading programs and organized their efforts in different ways. The parochial schools and one public school district had no reading specialists available to the students, and two public school districts had reading specialists in each elementary school building and at the junior high level. None of the schools offered diagnostic clinic reading services before the project, and most had no remedial programs involving a sizable number of students. Some of the schools did have developmental programs, which generally include special classes for groups of students and some individual work; however, this help was not offered on a uniform basis and was available in only two districts.

The special reading teachers in the districts had qualified for special certification through their own study programs and had attended various colleges and universities, often with different emphases in their approach to reading instruction. Some districts offered different programs in the various buildings within the district. Different texts were selected by building faculty in some cases. One district considered most reading problems chronic and therefore adopted one basic, comprehensive program with supplementary materials to lend continuity. The International Reading Association evaluation team recognized the program as outstanding.

The recent interest in the problem of reading has created many factions representing interested local groups, as well as some groups affiliated with national organizations. In addition, there are special parent groups that attempt to influence school programs in reading by applying pressure on faculty and school boards. Some parent groups are politically oriented and believe there is a Communist plot to make our schools ineffective, whereas others are influenced by professional groups, such as optometrists who offer inviting programs emphasizing their biases toward visual-perception training. Still other groups, such as the Learning Disabilities Association, join educators and the lay public in organizations designed to influence the school's offerings. Finally, industry, with kits to sell and programs to market, and a plethora of companies and practitioners, works at stirring up the climate around reading in the schools.

The educator is pressured by forces on the left and on the right. Some ask for a return to the McGuffey Readers, and others berate him for not having children crawl on the floor. Most competent educators are seeking proof in the literature for one program or another and find as many studies pointing one way as the other. At present, it would be safe to say that the literature does not contain evidence to justify the adoption of any particular program or approach.

Reading programs

Since there have been few studies that indicate conclusively the superiority of one method of instruction over another, and since, in addition, there is a strong possibility that individual learning problems may best be handled by varying methods, the training institutions for teachers usually offer different approaches to solving reading problems. The responsibility for securing education in the advanced reading programs is largely left to individual teachers, and therefore they attend many different colleges. It is likely that fifteen specialists in a district may represent as many schools of thought in reading instruction. Because comprehensive in-service training programs are lacking in most districts, it is extremely difficult to run programs that are well articulated and continuous. Since most reading problems are chronic and usually involve years of support, this can be a real problem.

A child who has a reading problem may be either educationally or physically handicapped; however, it is difficult to determine which is the actual cause of the reading disability. If it can be determined that the child has had inadequate instruction or that his problems began after reading instruction started, it might be assumed that he is educationally handicapped. If he can be given special instruction geared to the way he learns best, the prognosis is generally good. If, however, he has had adequate instruction involving various methods but still seems to be unable to read, we may have to admit that he probably will have a reading problem most of his life. One of the best indicators is an adequate history. Probably one or both of his parents and some of his siblings have reading problems. He will probably fail the Bender gestalt test if his problem is discovered early in his education, and he will have difficulty drawing a clock. He also will fail or have a low score on his Ortho-Rater examination and is likely to evidence behavior problems and later show some signs of depression.

Our program of diagnosis, like many others, is not costly, averaging $125 per client. Still, financing in the schools is difficult, and this cost does seem excessive to some when the entire yearly cost of educating a child averages about $700 in a suburban regular school. Furthermore, once the student's problem has been described and recommendations are made for treatment, the additional effort required to provide remediation includes the work of reading specialists or paraprofessionals who are not available.

Working with children in special intervention classes offers some solutions, not so much because of the immediate effect on the children but because the classes provide training for teachers and paraprofessionals in addition to serving as demonstration and research centers. The training should seek to establish some uniformity in program offerings so that the child will not change programs each time he changes teachers; however, it should also help teachers to appreciate many different approaches to remediation of reading problems.

Many programs also have the services of medical personnel who are interested in learning problems. Most of these medical personnel are in the fields of pediatric-neurology, psychiatry, and ophthalmology. Their involvement is usually the result of interest in the problem rather than the result of financial arrangements. They are not interested in finding sick children, because they are better able to do that in their own hospitals and because most suburban children rarely have significant medical problems not already being treated. In our project few of the children were found to be ill; few even needed glasses who did not already have them. About three children out of a thousand were discovered to have brain tumors, and two previously undetected cases of Huntington's chorea were found. There were many subtle deviations, however, that needed to be studied.

Each specialty will undoubtedly see different problems and must be willing to work through educators, both because of their time limitation and because of the educator's knowledge of what is possible in the school. This means that they must allow the practitioners in education to quarterback the treatment of reading problems.

Since there are many operational designs, it is neither possible, nor necessary for understanding, to elaborate on them. Instead I will list below the design of our program as a model of procedure you might expect to find in a public school reading clinic.

1. Initiation of the referral is by any of the following persons:
    a. Building principals
    b. Classroom teachers
    c. Guidance counselors
    d. Special reading teachers
    e. Parents
2. All referrals must be approved by the building principal and the district reading supervisor. (This structure is used, first, to ensure the cooperation of the principal when a program is recommended for the child, and, second, to ensure that the child has been given all the help the regular program can offer before being referred to the clinic. Where the clinics can handle only a limited number of clients, it also serves to order the cases according to the seriousness of the problems.)
3. The school referral is then sent to the reading clinic.
4. The clinic staff either accepts or rejects the referral on the basis of the information on the referral form. This information includes the following:
    a. Reasons for referral
    b. Description of school behavior
    c. Past test results from the student's individual student record
    d. Health information
5. After the referral has been accepted by the reading clinic, the school is notified in writing that the child has been accepted.
6. The school then notifies the parents of the referral.
7. After a short waiting period, long enough for the school to notify the parents, the parents are sent a form letter asking them to call the clinic for an appointment for both parents and the child.
8. Appointments are made for two sessions.
    a. *First session*

        (1) Parents interviewed by reading specialist or guidance counselor

        (2) Client administered the following tests:

            (a) Durrell Analysis of Reading Difficulty

            (b) Fifty words from the Dolch Basic Sight Word Test

            (c) Interest inventory

    b. *Second session*

        (1) Child administered Wechsler Intelligence Scale for Children (WISC) by reading specialists or guidance counselor

        (2) After administration of WISC, child given the following tests:

            (a) Burnett Reading Series: Survey Test

            (b) Nonstandardized word recognition skills test

            (c) Any other tests that seem appropriate: Wepman's Auditory Discrimination Test; the Bender gestalt test; the Peabody Picture Vocabulary Test; and the Memory-for-Designs Test

9. The child is given a pediatric screening by the clinic medical staff. During the screening, the child's vision and hearing are checked by members of the clinic staff.

10. Any member of the staff can refer the child to the center's neurologist, psychologist, psychiatrist, or ophthalmologist.

11. After all the testing has been completed, the clinicians involved in the case make a case report, with a reading specialist being in charge.

The case report is then sent to the school. The parents are notified by letter that the study has been completed and that specific recommendations have been sent to the school. The letter also briefly summarizes the findings of the clinic.

We have found in the last year that we have had to develop an exit interview for parents after the completion of the study because of their anxiety. There is a problem of helping parents accept the limitations of our schools in handling problems that do not respond to the regular-school reading program. It has also been found wise to have an educator conduct the exit interview, because he is able to help the parents understand disagreements among consultants and to gain their cooperation in the program.

After a period of six months, the parents are asked to respond to the behavioral checklist to which they responded during their first interview. The list is analyzed along with other data from the school and retesting to assess the program's progress.

The identification of those children who are unlikely to respond to support programs is difficult. One of our frequent recommendations is to work with the child's assets whenever possible. Another is to accept a wider behavior pattern while working with deficits, being very sensitive to the frustration level of the child.

The program recommended to the school and family is outlined in great detail, and when recommendations are made, they are the result of a comprehensive study of the facilities of the school as well as the abilities of the faculty and child. The recommendations, therefore, are made within the framework of what is possible in a specific setting and with the recognition that the recommendation of limited change is better than a comprehensive recommendation that cannot be implemented. As a rule, various levels of help are recommended in case more help becomes available. Although the recommendations are directed toward the present setting and resources, the clinic staff continually studies the needs of the child to help effect future changes in developing reading programs in the schools that will be more effective each year. Thus the development of programs based on accumulated evidence rather than on commercially produced programs and publicity-generated fads is also a by-product of the interdisciplinary approach.

Development of this type of program must be slow and at times turbulent. Overly rapid expansion due to popularity plagues such programs as much as the roadblocks constructed by groups of professionals who feel that their territorial prerogatives are threatened and the financial barriers that accompany any educational enterprise in our society. Too rapid expansion can result in an ineffective program because of improperly trained personnel and the use of poor tools and techniques.

Case studies

Most educators have great difficulty in applying the term "dyslexia." This stems from an inability to diagnose a case without first knowing that the client is unable to read. Although recognizing this, some physicians choose to use the term because they have found that when they do, the school stops its effort to teach the child, thus relieving the pressures on the child.

This approach does work in many cases, and possibly in most cases. However, educators offering comprehensive programs of diagnosis and remediation resent the diagnosis. The major problem is that if a child does not read in our schools, he is offered no alternate curriculum. There is no "bookless curriculum" at present. Instead, a child is passed on, or in some schools placed in a program geared primarily to mildly retarded children. In most cases it is hoped that the child can survive to be admitted into a vocational program. Unfortunately, such programs are not geared to children with reading disability, either.

At this point four case reports can be examined in detail. I have selected case reports that can serve to illustrate the type of problem we have been discussing as dyslexia, or whatever you might choose to call it.

CASE B

Birth date 9/20/60   Grade 2   Seen during first period

I. GENERAL OBSERVATIONS

B was accompanied to all testing sessions by his mother. He was relaxed during the interview and testing sessions, and related well with the examiner.

SCHOOL REFERRAL: B does not recognize most of the letters of the alphabet and is unable to recall more than a few words. He seems to be interested in attending the special reading class and is always prompt. He does not seem interested in putting

---

Continued.

CASE B—cont'd

forth a great deal of effort but is enthusiastic about any of his accomplishments (experience stories and kinesthetic approach).

PARENT INTERVIEW: An interview with the mother was conducted by the reading clinic's guidance counselor. The mother said that B does not know all his ABC's, and his grades are down in reading and spelling. She feels that he has a poor memory for schoolwork. The mother feels that the child had a bad experience in grade 1. The mother claims that B knew his ABC's in kindergarten but regressed during the first grade experience. This year (1968-1969) he likes his teacher and his conduct has improved.

The mother reports that B is her child by a previous marriage. He has not been legally adopted by her present husband but goes by his name, considers him his father, and is unaware that he has a natural father somewhere. The parents plan to tell B "gradually" that Mr. W is his stepfather.

The mother says that B is not close to his stepfather because he is not an easy person to get close to or understand. He guards his privacy closely and wants no one to intrude, including his wife and children. The stepfather does little with B. The mother says she is fairly close to B but that he sometimes keeps problems from her.

The mother said that B has no close friends. He is interested in being a cub scout. He is basically a follower but is not easily led.

II. PHYSICAL ASSESSMENT

PEDIATRIC EXAMINATION: A pediatric physical examination was conducted by the center's medical staff. This examination revealed no educationally significant abnormalities.

VISION: B's vision was checked by a member of the reading staff using the Bausch & Lomb Ortho-Rater. All responses were in the normal range.

HEARING: The center's hearing clinician checked B's hearing with a full-scale audiogram on the Miniature E. B. Audiometer, model 60. All responses were good.

NOTE: The neurologist gave the following information not included in the report: Marked latency and hesitancy in *all* responses that he is unable to do—mild diffuse spasticity, developmental. Pleasant lad with marked symbolic language disorder, including symbolic recall and phasic verbal expression, mild spasticity and clumsiness, developmental and probably constitutional.

III. TEST DATA

A brief inventory of interests was used to put B at ease while finding out something about his interests and attitudes. He said that he likes to play with his brother and sister and watch television in his spare time. B does not belong to any clubs or organizations, nor does he have a hobby. He stated that he likes school with arithmetic being his favorite subject. He said that he likes to have someone read to him.

DOLCH BASIC SIGHT WORD TEST: A 50-word sample of the Dolch list of 220 basic words was used to check sight vocabulary. B was unable to respond to any of the words.

DURRELL ANALYSIS OF READING DIFFICULTY: This individually administered battery of reading tests was given with the following results:

Oral and silent reading: B was unable to do either of these subtests because of his inability to read the material.

Listening comprehension: Listening comprehension was adequate at the third grade level.

Letters named: This subtest was administered to determine B's knowledge of the alphabet. In naming capital letters he missed 10 out of 26; on the lower case letters he missed 13 out of 26.

CASE B—cont'd

Visual memory of words—primary: B was able to remember 7 out of 20 words flashed to him. This performance is below test norms.

Hearing sounds in words: This subtest is given to children who cannot perform the "hearing sounds in words—primary" test because they do not know the alphabet. It helps to discover the severity of the difficulty in perception of sounds in words. B was able to discriminate the specific sounds of "m," "s," and "f" adequately.

Learning rate: This test is designed primarily for the nonreader or the preprimer reader. Its purpose is to discover the degree of difficulty the child has in remembering words taught. Five words were taught. After an interval of about 30 minutes, B was able to remember 2 of 5 words.

WEPMAN AUDITORY DISCRIMINATION TEST: Given to determine whether B has an auditory discrimination problem, this test indicated inadequate discrimination development, with B missing 9 pairs of words. The maximum number of errors in the normal range for his age level is 3.

READING READINESS: The reading-readiness section of a nonstandardized test was administered to check B's visual and auditory discrimination. This test indicated that B has the ability to visually discriminate between groups of words. He showed an inadequacy in auditory discrimination.

INTELLIGENCE TEST: The Wechsler Intelligence Scale for Children was administered and the following scores were obtained:

 Verbal IQ = 81   *Performance IQ = 90*   *Full-scale IQ = 84*

Examiner's note: B is inclined to give a long pause or no response; he resists saying he does not know, but guesses. The child may not be particularly alert to his environment, especially to facts and details. He may very well be in an environment that has not been intellectually stimulating.

IV. SUMMARY AND RECOMMENDATIONS

TEST RESULTS: B was pleasant and cooperative in the clinical setting, and test results confirm that his mental abilities are in the dull-normal range. An IQ of 84, coupled with his second grade placement, indicates that he should be reading at about a low first grade level. However, he is actually functioning below his expectancy level.

The Durrell Analysis and Dolch's Basic Sight Word Test both confirmed that B does not have a sight vocabulary. He was unable to respond to any word on either test.

Test results indicate that B is deficient in most skills needed for reading. He does not know the alphabet, he does not have a sight vocabulary, and he has poor auditory discrimination. These skills need to be developed before serious reading instruction can begin.

RECOMMENDED INSTRUCTION: Instruction should begin with the recognition of letters of the alphabet and their appropriate sounds in isolated form and within words. After B has learned the alphabet, work should begin in auditory discrimination. The following technique could be used in developing auditory discrimination:

1. Provide a list of spoken words containing the element to be taught.
2. Have B focus his attention on that particular sound in the words.
3. Have him compare words that contain the sound with words that do not.
4. Encourage him to think of additional words that contain the sound.

After B has developed auditory discrimination skills, work could begin on word analysis skills. At the same time, instruction in sight vocabulary could begin. To develop word meaning, as well as sight vocabulary, the words should be presented in context.

Basal group instruction within the classroom should be on a beginning preprimer

Continued.

CASE B—cont'd

level. Although B may have been taken through the preprimers, he did not acquire the skills presented.

OTHER POSSIBLE TESTS: Since B has not learned in the present situation, a new approach might be tried. In teaching sight words, the tactile approach could be used. This is a long, drawn-out process, but it could be helpful in teaching B to read. Using this approach, have B trace and vocalize the sounds of the letters. These sounds must be blended simultaneously with the letters being traced. After tracing and blending the sounds several times, ask him to close his eyes and print the word in the air as he sounds the word aloud. This tactile approach is suggested in daily usage of ten minutes at a time. This method was used in the clinic in teaching B the word "that." He was able to remember the word after a two-hour interval. Some individualized teaching will be required to implement the teaching techniques and materials suggested. B can best be helped if a remedial reading teacher takes him from the classroom for individual instruction.

PROGNOSIS: The prognosis in B's case does not appear to be bright. Because his intelligence score falls in the dull-normal range, and because he has spent two years in reading instruction without success, a long-range supportive program will have to be provided to improve his reading achievement.

MATERIALS: The following materials could be helpful in remediating B's reading problem:

1. Basal reading program (for example, Scott-Foresman's Starter Concept Cards, Ready to Roll, Rolling Along)
2. Scott-Foresman's Talking Alphabet, Parts I and II
3. Dolch's Basic Sight Vocabulary Cards
4. Linguistic Block Series (Scott-Foresman)
5. Working With Sounds, Book A (Barnell Loft)
6. Phonics We Use (Lyons & Carnahan)
7. Phonics Workbook, Grade I (Modern Curriculum Press)
8. Time for Phonics, Book A (McGraw-Hill Book Co.)
9. Starting Phonics, Grade I (Milliken Publishers)

I have selected the case reports for this section to illustrate the progressive use of the recommendations of the various disciplines by the educators. In the case of B, above, the educator chose to ignore the observations of the neurologist entirely, because he was unable to fit them into his frame of reference. This was an early case for the worker in the project. In the case report on P, below, the educator uses the neurologist's observations but makes no attempt to incorporate them into his recommendations.

CASE P

Birth date 12/27/60   Grade 1

I. GENERAL OBSERVATIONS

P was accompanied to the center by his parents. He was fairly relaxed during the interview and testing sessions, and related well with the examiner.

SCHOOL REFERRAL: Background forms were filled out by the home and school.

CASE P—cont'd

They disclosed that P had been retained in the first grade. The school referral stated that P has difficulty in remembering: "One day he knows a word, and the next day he has no idea what the same word is."

PARENT INTERVIEW: The parent interview was conducted by the counselor from the reading clinic. The parents first noted P's reading problem about midway through the first grade. They said P was unable to assoicate letters and sounds with words. The parents feel he is learning his beginning sounds now and is improving in his reading. During the interview, the mother indicated that she had had difficulty in learning reading and also that their second child had a reading problem. The mother sees P as a normal child, somewhat smaller than other children. She also stated that he tends to be a "follower" rather than a "leader." The parents do not view P as a discipline problem. They feel that he is accepted well by both his peers and adults. The parents insist that P complete college, but they do not expect him to make above-average grades in school.

II. PHYSICAL ASSESSMENT

PEDIATRIC EXAMINATION: P was given a pediatric physical examination by the center's medical staff. The pediatrician did not find any abnormalities in his examination except that P is small for his age and has moderate caries. It is suggested that P see his dentist.

NEUROLOGICAL EXAMINATION: P was given a neurological examination by the center's neurologist. The neurologist described it as a normal neurological examination except that P has a small head. P was diagnosed as having very low phonetic language development, with low verbal expression ability and low tactile cortical responses. He was described as having good coordination, with no abnormal movements. He is right-handed, right-eyed, and right-footed, without any confusion. There are indications of a family history of reading and spelling difficulties. The neurologist diagnoses P as having a mild-to-moderate reading problem on a constitutional basis. The neurologist would like to reexamine P in one year. The neurologist recommends that P be referred to the Central Institute for the Deaf for a language evaluation.

VISION: Vision was checked by a member of the center's staff using the Bausch & Lomb Ortho-Rater. This examination indicates a possible deficiency in far-point acuity in both the right and left eyes, as well as a complete deficiency in near-point acuity. P was referred to the center's ophthalmologist for further examination. This examination revealed that P has 20/20 vision in each eye and no ocular pathology. Testing of visual skills resulted in an almost perfect score. Visual-perception testing showed reversals and confusion in direction but normal perception of size relationships.

HEARING: Hearing was checked by the hearing consultant with a full-scale audiogram on the Miniature E. B. Audiometer. All responses were good.

III. TEST DATA

DURRELL ANALYSIS OF READING DIFFICULTY: This individually administered battery of reading tests was given with the following results:

Oral reading: P was asked to read paragraphs at levels 1 and 2. On paragraph 1, P made 8 errors, with 75% comprehension; therefore a basal level could not be established. On paragraph 2, P made 26 errors, with 67% comprehension; the time was 3 minutes, 56 seconds, which is well beyond the acceptable time limit of 2 minutes. P is a word-by-word reader with a short eye span. He has a very low sight vocabulary and does not appear to have the ability to use word-analysis skills.

Continued.

CASE P—cont'd

Silent reading: P was asked to read paragraph 1. He was unable to recall anything about the story, with the exception of the name "Peter." On direct questions of the material, P was unable to respond to any of the questions. From this performance, it appears that P has such a low sight vocabulary that he was unable to comprehend what he had read.

Listening comprehension: Listening was adequate at the grade 2 level.

Word recognition and word analysis: Word recognition resulted in 7 out of 19 of the grade 1 reading level, list A. In word analysis, P was able to improve by only 1 word. Both these performances would place P at a low first grade level.

Letters named: P was given this subtest and made the following errors:

Capital letters—called J-G, V-Y, and N-M

Lower case letters—called t-g, j-g, l-i, y-n, b-y, and q-p

Visual memory of words—primary: P was able to remember the letters and words long enough to circle 10 out of 20. This performance is below test norms.

Hearing sounds in words—primary: P was able to distinguish the sounds in words for a score of 14 out of 29. His performance was very poor on beginning consonant blends, sound endings, and the combination of beginning and ending sounds. This performance is below test norms.

Spelling: P was able to spell only 1 word correctly (look). This performance is below test norms.

INTELLIGENCE TEST: The Wechsler Intelligence Scale for Children was administered by the center's psychometrist, with the following results:

Verbal IQ = 109   Performance IQ = 108   Full-scale IQ = 109

WIDE RANGE ACHIEVEMENT TEST: This test was administered with the following results:

	GRADE PLACEMENT	PERCENTILE
Reading	1.4	10
Spelling	1.4	10
Arithmetic	2.1	27

PEABODY PICTURE VOCABULARY TEST: This was administered with the following results:

MA = 7-3   IQ = 93   Percentile = 36

IV. SUMMARY AND RECOMMENDATIONS

PHYSICAL ASSESSMENT: P appeared to be a healthy 7-year-old Caucasian male. He was pleasant and cooperative in the clinical setting, and test results confirmed that his mental abilities are within the normal range. P's reading problem is great enough to warrant any corrective help that can be provided.

The neurological and pediatric examinations revealed that P has moderate caries and that he should be referred to a dentist. It is recommended that P be given a neurological reexamination in August, 1969. It is also recommended that P be given a language evaluation by the Central Institute for the Deaf.

P has been referred to the center's ophthalmology consultant for a thorough eye examination. This examination revealed that P has 20/20 vision in each eye and no ocular pathology.

TEST RESULTS: The Durrell Analysis indicates that P is deficient in most of the skills needed for reading. He was unable to name some letters of the alphabet. This deficiency would make it very difficult for P to use phonics in word analysis. Because he does not know some of the letters and their appropriate sounds, he would not be able to analyze a word that contained any of these unknown letters. P's sight vocabulary, which is so necessary at this level, is low. Because he does not know some

CASE P—cont'd

letters of the alphabet, is deficient in word analysis skills, and has a low sight vocabulary, P was unable to read the first grade paragraphs. This indicates that his instructional reading level is below the first grade level. Since his instructional level is so low, P does not have an independent reading level. Since he does not have an independent reading level, P would not be able to build a sight vocabulary by reading independently. With these deficiencies, P's comprehension is low because he is unable to use context clues to help him understand what he reads. Therefore it is of utmost importance to correct these deficiencies.

On the Hearing Sounds in Words, a subtest of the Durrell Analysis, P's performance was below test norms. He was able to use beginning sounds fairly well, scoring 6 out of 7 correctly. He did poorly in hearing beginning consonant blends and consonant digraphs, identifying 3 out of 8 correctly. He missed all the words on ending sounds. On the section involving a combination of hearing beginning and ending sounds, he was able to identify only 3 out of 8 correctly. These results indicate that P is able to use only beginning consonant sounds and is almost completely unable to hear other sounds in a word.

PROGNOSIS: Based on the findings of this clinic, the prognosis in P's case does not appear to be too bright. P was almost 7 years old (December birthday) when he entered the first grade. At this age and with a high normal intelligence, he should have been able to grasp first grade material without much difficulty. However, he was not able to do so. Presently, P is a first grader, almost 8 years old, who still lacks the skills needed to successfully perform at a first grade level.

RECOMMENDED INSTRUCTION: The following recommendations concerning instruction are made:

1. P should receive instruction in recognition of letters of the alphabet and their appropriate sounds in isolated form and within words.

2. P's sight vocabulary needs to be increased. This could be done by using Dolch's Basic Sight Vocabulary Cards or any other material designed for sight vocabulary building.

3. P needs instruction in hearing sounds in words, especially beginning consonant blends and digraphs, and ending sounds. Materials such as Consonant Lotto and/or any similar material available to the school would be useful in remediating this particular problem.

4. After P has mastered the letters of the alphabet and is able to hear sounds in words, he should receive intensive instruction in word analysis.

5. The above suggestions may be incorporated into P's regular reading program or into a remedial or clinical setting.

6. If P is placed in a regular reading program, it is recommended that beginning first grade material be used. He should be kept at each instructional level of this program until he has successfully mastered the skills involved. This type of instruction may be necessary for P's entire elementary-school life. It is expected that with proper instruction and good use of materials, P's reading problem can be alleviated.

MATERIALS: The following materials are recommended:

1. Basic reading program (Scott-Foresman's Starter Concept Cards, Ready to Roll, Rolling Along)
2. The Talking Alphabet, Parts I and II, to instruct P in hearing sounds in words
3. Dolch's Basic Sight Vocabulary Cards or other materials of this type for improving P's sight vocabulary
4. Benefic Press's Interest and Low Vocabulary Series, such as The Button Family Series and The Cowboy Sam Series, both at pre-primer level (may be helpful in building P's sight vocabulary and comprehension)

The case report of S, below, illustrates how the clinician incorporates the recommendation of the neurologist into his report and into the final recommendations. This case report is one of those more recently seen by the clinic.

CASE S

Birth date 1/25/57   Grade 7

I.   REASON FOR REFERRAL

Reading, spelling, homework, and vocabulary are below normal levels. S experiences difficulty in recognizing words, understanding what he reads, and spelling.

II.   TEST DATA

DOLCH BASIC SIGHT WORD TEST: A 50-word sample of the Dolch list of 220 basic service words was used to check sight vocabulary. S supplied 49 of these words immediately. This performance would place him at approximately the third grade level.

DURRELL ANALYSIS OF READING DIFFICULTY: This individually administered battery of reading tests was given with the following results:

Oral reading: S was asked to read paragraphs at grade levels 3, 4, and 5. A basic reading level was reached at the third grade level. He had some difficulty with paragraph 4, and reached a frustration level on paragraph 5. He reads with a monotonous tone and uses incorrect phrasing.

Silent reading: S was asked to read paragraphs at grade levels 3 and 4. He had very good unaided recall (comprehension) on both paragraphs. He had a tendency to omit specific details, but otherwise, his recall was well organized and comprehensive.

Listening comprehension: This skill is adequate at the sixth grade level. The fact that S was unable to understand material read to him above a sixth grade level is significant because of his seventh grade placement.

Word recognition and word analysis: S was able to recognize 31 of the 50 words flashed to him from the grade 2-6 reading level. This performance would place him at a high fourth grade level. When he was given time to analyze the words he missed when they were flashed, he was able to pronounce 6 additional words. This gain is not sufficient to assume good word analysis skills. The gain could be due to sight vocabulary.

Visual memory of words—intermediate: Five of 15 words flashed to S were remembered long enough for him to write them correctly. This performance is at the fourth grade level. A student in the seventh grade should be able to remember at least 10 of the 15 words.

Hearing sounds in words: This performance was below test norms, with 4 of 15 polysyllabic words spelled consistently from a sounding standpoint. This would indicate inadequate phonic skills.

Spelling: S was able to spell 5 of the 20 words from the grade 4 and above list. This performance is below test norms, which show that a score of 6 correct words would place him at the third grade level.

BURNETT READING SERIES: SURVEY TEST (INTERMEDIATE): This standardized silent reading test was given with the following results:

CASE S—cont'd

SUBTEST	PERCENTILE (based on 6.8 grade norms)
Word identification	1
Word meaning	1
Comprehension	1
Total survey	1
Grade equivalency	3.4

INTELLIGENCE TEST: The Wechsler Intelligence Scale for Children was administered, and the following scores were obtained:

Verbal IQ = 94   Performance IQ = 118   Full-scale IQ = 106

III. PHYSICAL ASSESSMENT

VISION: S's vision was checked by means of a Bausch & Lomb Ortho-Rater. All
responses were in the normal range.

HEARING: The center's hearing clinician checked S's hearing, using the E. B.
Miniature Audiometer, model 60. All responses were good except at 6,000 decibels,
which is not significant.

NEUROLOGICAL SCREENING: S was examined by the center's consulting neurologist.
He found S to have poor sequential memory, almost nonexistent symbolic recall, and
a global symbolic language disorder. The neurologist made the following recommendations:

1. Regular school, with the following:
   a. Continuous matriculation
   b. Special considerations with reference to S's poor symbolic language dis-
      order
2. In reference to 1b: use of television, tapes, lectures, and objective tests such
   as true-false, multiple choice, and yes-no as much as possible.

IV. SUMMARY AND RECOMMENDATIONS

TEST RESULTS: S was pleasant and cooperative in the clinical setting, and test
results confirmed that his present level of intellectual functioning is in the normal
range. An IQ of 106, coupled with his seventh grade placement, would indicate that
he should have been reading at about the beginning eighth grade level at the time
of his testing. However, S is actually functioning at a fourth grade level. His reading
problem is great enough to warrant any corrective help that can be provided.

S's sight vocabulary appears to be at a high fourth grade level. His word analysis
skills include consistency in the use of initial consonant blends, consonant digraphs,
and ending sounds. He has some difficulty and is inconsistent in regard to vowel
sounds and syllables in the medial positions. Materials such as Lyons and Carnahan's
Phonics We Use and McGraw-Hill's *Conquests in Reading* would provide the necessary drills to improve his word analysis skills. These publications provide a variety
of drills in phonetic analysis, syllabication, and other word analysis skills. If S is
able to improve his word analysis skills, his overall reading performance should
improve. These skills would allow him to attack unknown words, he would become
more proficient in using a dictionary, and his overall reading fluency would be increased. At the present time, it is necessary for him to seek help when he comes to
an unknown word, or to skip over it, which is probably what happens most often.
Thus his reading continuity is broken and his comprehension suffers.

RECOMMENDED INSTRUCTION: It will be necessary for S's teachers to adjust their
expectations of his overall performance. At the present time, it is very improbable

Continued.

CASE S—cont'd

that S can read and understand material at his present grade level. Reading assignments should be kept at a minimum or, if possible, discontinued. Since he is unable to read without frustration, the educational value of reading assignments will be almost, if not completely, nonexistent.

S could probably profit from a vocational-technical education whenever it becomes available. He appears to be interested in this area, and his test scores indicate that his talent would lie in that direction. His major weakness is in the area of language, around which the academic curriculum is built; therefore, areas of the curriculum that are not language oriented would probably be best for S.

PROGNOSIS: S's prognosis does not appear to be good. His neurological shortcomings will hamper him in the academic–college-preparatory type of curriculum. However, the global language disorder should not keep him from being a resourceful citizen after he completes his education. It will probably be necessary for the school to adopt a course of study that will be within S's functioning ability.

A parent conference with Mrs. E was conducted in April, 1970.

A final illustrative case report concerns a dyslexic boy who was one of the first to be seen by the project reading clinic. The first write-up was completed by a group of clinicians who rejected the consultant's views; the comments of the consultant are included. Later, because the child's problems continued, he was reexamined and an addendum report was issued. The clinician who wrote the first report left the program because of an inability to function within the multidisciplinary setting. I realize that this is a biased view because of my involvement in the dispute, and I wish to emphasize this so that the reader can draw his own conclusion. The boy's problem has continued, and he has dropped out of school. At present he is unable to find schooling even through vocational training. The problem is clearly one of dyslexia—extreme reading disability—and is present also in most of his siblings.

CASE D

Birth date 2/27/54   Grade 8 (not in school now)

I. BACKGROUND

SCHOOL REFERRAL: D was referred because of a reading disability. The teachers describe his behavior as cooperative and friendly.

CUMULATIVE RECORD: September, 1966—S.R.A.: Achievement-Reading 13th percentile

July, 1966   WISC   Full-scale IQ = 97

OTHER AGENCIES: Child guidance clinic, July 18, 1966; Special school district, March 1, 1966.

CASE D—cont'd

II. SENSORY SCREENING

VISION: The Bausch & Lomb Ortho-Rater Occupational and School Vision Tests indicated adequate usable vision without glasses.

HEARING: A hearing test was administered by means of the E. B. Miniature Audiometer, model 60. D failed the 30-decibel sweep check test (left ear at high frequency). It was recommended that he have another screening test in six months.

III. PSYCHOLOGICAL ASSESSMENT

WECHSLER INTELLIGENCE SCALE FOR CHILDREN:

VERBAL TESTS		PERFORMANCE TESTS	
Information	6	Picture completion	10
Comprehension	9	Picture arrangement	10
Arithmetic	4	Block design	11
Similarities	9	Object assembly	14
Vocabulary	8	Coding	11
(Digit span)	11		

Verbal IQ = 82   Performance IQ = 108   Full-scale IQ = 94

IV. EDUCATIONAL ASSESSMENT

DURRELL ANALYSIS OF READING DIFFICULTY:

	GRADE EQUIVALENT
Word recognition	2.9
Word analysis	3.5
Instructional level	2.1
Independent level	1.2
Expectancy level	7.1

WIDE RANGE ACHIEVEMENT TEST (revised edition, 1965):

	GRADE	STANDARD SCORE	PERCENTILE
Reading	2.6	66	1
Spelling	2.6	66	1
Arithmetic	2.3	64	1

The only words that D could spell correctly on the test were "eat" and "run." D then attempted 28 more words on the list without evidencing any anxiety or tension. He simply wrote the words as if he knew exactly how to spell them correctly. However, there was no apparent logic in the spelling; there were very few phonetic correlations between sound and symbol within the words. In almost all the words, though, the first letter was correct, and almost as many were spelled with the correct letter at the end.

On the reading test, D's attempts to figure out the words that were difficult for him usually resulted in his substituting words of similar configuration. Some reversals were evident, particularly where there was an "r" and vowel combination. He also sometimes reversed whole syllables within a word.

On the arithmetic test, D seemed unable to solve even the simpler addition and subtraction problems, and he was not able to do any long division. He attempted some multiplication and some fraction problems but was unsuccessful. He attempted one square root problem and was successful.

Continued.

CASE D—cont'd

EVALUATION OF SPEECH AND LANGUAGE SKILLS: On Wepman's Auditory Discrimination Test there are indications that D has difficulty in attending to speech sounds. This does not involve his hearing acuity, which is normal within the speech frequencies.

V. CONSULTING STAFF

PEDIATRICIAN: The physical examination of this boy is not remarkable: height, 64¼ inches; weight, 108 pounds; urine, negative; blood pressure, 116 over 52. He is a well-nourished preadolescent lad who is cooperative, friendly, and pleasant.

NEUROLOGIST: This 13-year 9-month-old adolescent white male demonstrates many mild but definite neurological handicaps. The etiology is unclear but is probably congenital—possibly related to the pregnancy but more likely constitutional and familial. The neurological disability is manifested by gross motor incoordination, especially of the large muscles of the upper and lower extremities (although there is fairly adequate fine digit control); excessive mirror and associative movements; mild spasticity in the lower extremities, with hyperactive deep tendon reflexes (left greater than right); and bilateral functional metatarsus varus more on the left than on the right, with a toeing-in, toe-walking type of gait associated with immature language development at the higher cortical level. Mild expressive dysphasia is present, along with difficulty with body image and spatial relations. His speech is also handicapped by a motor disarticulation problem. I could elicit no visual-perceptual, visual-memory, or visual-motor problem, even though this youngster states that information presented geometrically and visually is difficult for him to understand. His strengths appear to be his auditory receptive mechanism and manual activity (other than large motor activity). This youngster also demonstrates a type of cognitive disability in regard to stored information, the concept of time, and general language development. His judgment is tenuous. He wishes to please and attempted all the tasks with much vigor; yet minor sullen behavior was evident on occasion, and he might be overly suggestible.

Consultant note: This is not adequate copying of my interpretation: dyslexia, with a severe symbolic language problem, *is* the major problem.

PSYCHOLOGIST: The personality testing and projectives show that D demonstrates a considerable amount of anxiety and feeling of inferiority, with concern about his achievement on the test, but more generally a sense of defeat in life. Even beforehand he feels that he cannot achieve. He expresses his unsureness and inadequacy by saying: "Well, it's sort of . . .," or "It could be," or "That's strange." But he also creates the inadequate forms for his inadequate percepts by a certain amount of what is called confabulation—that is, he creates a good and accurate percept and then extends it to an inaccurate area. This is partly an expression of a lack of a sense of reality, but this lack is based on manifest anxiety and a need to deal with anxiety in social relations by distorting reality. He tries to patch over his anxiety by being safe, by describing rather than interpreting, and also by distorting. He verbalizes his awareness of his inadequacy.

More particularly however, there is an anxiety about belonging—where, and to whom. He wonders how strange, weird, ugly, and different he is. He feels he does not belong. He feels unlucky but also has some guilt feeling that he is responsible for his ill luck—that is, he does not feel safe about attributing the luck or the unluckiness to anybody else. He feels he is floating and detached from the whole but denies any coherent sense of the whole and what place there might be in it for him. Things are out of focus—upside down, distorted—but his own efforts, minimal as they are, do not seem to right them, and he gives up. There is much self-defeat.

CASE D—cont'd

VI. CLINIC STAFFING RECOMMENDATIONS

EDUCATIONAL:

1. It is recommended that D and his parents renew their relationship with the university clinic.
2. The school should keep in mind that until the family secures psychotherapy, little academic progress is likely; however, the following recommendations might be tried by the reading teacher, realizing that, developmentally, D is ready for reading instruction on a beginning second grade level.
   a. Word analysis should be taught only in context and should not be used in isolation drill. Further, the skills should be taught only as the need for them arises. However, D does need some work with digraphs and final consonants to help correct his inaccurate analysis. He also needs work in recognizing diphthongs and their sounds.
   b. Structural analysis also needs emphasis but, again, only in context. D should learn to note endings, prefixes, and suffixes, and to separate words into known parts.
   c. D needs to learn to use context clues to correct his faulty analysis and to anticipate the unknown word.
   d. Easy reading on a first grade level needs to be done to improve phrasing and sight vocabulary. D should read as much as possible both at home and at school.
   e. A basic sight vocabulary needs to be developed, but this will probably have to be done with auditory reinforcement due to poor visual memory. The Language Master or the Programmed Reading series (Buchanan and Sullivan) would be very good for this purpose.

Consultant note: I disagree with this nonsense. My impression is that the problem is severe dyslexia in a nice, dependent, highly motivated lad who has difficulty in all areas of symbolic language.

HOME: It is felt that the recommendations made by the university child guidance clinic were adequate interpretations of the situation and that the severity of the problem should be emphasized and confirmed to the parents. This is not simply a reading—academic—difficulty. It is a generalized personality problem—not only D's but his parents' as well.

VII. ADDENDUM REPORT

D returned to the clinic for a follow-up neurological examination. At that time, the neurologist suggested a reevaluation of D's reading ability. An appointment was made for a testing session to examine his reading problem. In this session, the Dolch Basic Sight Word Test, the Durrell Analysis of Reading Difficulty, and the Burnett Reading Series: Survey Test were administered. The following are the results of these tests and the recommendations:

DOLCH SIGHT WORDS: The Dolch list of 220 basic sight words was used to check D's sight vocabulary. He was able to pronounce 187 of these words immediately. Normally, a pupil reading comfortably at a third grade level would respond immediately and accurately to all the words.

DURRELL ANALYSIS OF READING DIFFICULTY: This individually administered battery of reading tests was administered with the following results:

Oral reading: D was asked to read paragraphs at grade levels 2, 3, and 4. A basal level was reached at the level 2 paragraph, where he had no reading errors and 100% comprehension. On the level 3 paragraph, he had 1 reading error and

Continued.

CASE D—cont'd

100% comprehension. A breakdown in reading fluency occurred on paragraph 4, where D made 13 reading errors.

Silent reading: D was asked to read paragraphs 2, 3, and 4. D's reading comprehension was adequate on paragraphs 2 and 3, with a complete breakdown in comprehension on paragraph 4. There was constant lip movement and some whispering while D was reading silently.

Listening comprehension: D was read paragraphs above sixth grade level, at sixth grade level, and at fifth grade level. His listening comprehension was inadequate both above and at sixth grade level. Comprehension was adequate at the fifth grade level, indicating that he would have difficulty understanding material read to him above a fifth grade level.

Word recognition and word analysis: D was able to recognize 13 out of 39 words flashed to him, placing him at a middle third grade level. When given time to analyze the words he missed when they were flashed, he was able to improve his word recognition by 6 words, placing him at a low third grade level.

Visual memory of words—primary: D was able to remember 16 out of 20 words flashed to him. This performance would place him at a middle second grade level.

Hearing sounds in words—primary: D scored 27 out of 29 on this subtest. This performance is near the middle third grade level.

Visual memory of words—intermediate: D was able to remember 1 out of 15 words flashed to him. This performance is below test norms.

Phonic spelling of words: D's performance was below test norms, with none of the 15 polysyllabic words spelled consistently from a sounding standpoint. There were no consistencies in the use of beginning and ending syllables.

Spelling test: On the list of grade 4 and above, D's performance was below test norms.

BURNETT READING SERIES: SURVEY TEST (ADVANCED): This standardized silent reading test was administered with the following results:

	RAW SCORE	PERCENTILE
Word meaning	9	6
Rate and accuracy	3	Below norms
Comprehension	12	Below norms
Total survey	21	Below norms

VIII. SUMMARY AND RECOMMENDATIONS

TEST RESULTS: D was cooperative during the testing session and responded well with the examiner. On a WISC, administered in October, 1967, D obtained a full-scale score of 94.

Although placed in eighth grade, D's instructional level in reading appears to be about third grade level, based on the results of the Durrell Analysis of Reading Difficulty. He appears to rely solely on his sight vocabulary (words instantly recognized), which is at the third grade level, and has consistent use of beginning consonant sounds. Beyond this, he appears without any real word-attack skills when it comes to pronouncing a word he has not previously met in his reading.

It is evident from the Durrell Analysis that any reading above the third grade level is frustrating for D. His reading fluency and comprehension are very adequate at the third grade level, even though his reading speed is at a second grade level. A complete breakdown in both fluency and comprehension occurred when he tried to read paragraphs at the fourth grade level.

CASE D—cont'd

Normally a person is able to comprehend material read to him above his grade level. This was not so in D's case. The examiner had to drop back to a fifth grade level before D was able to comprehend adequately. From an educational viewpoint, this is a very serious problem. It appears that D is unable to understand material read to him at his grade level. Therefore, presenting material to D orally is not the solution to his educational problem.

RECOMMENDED INSTRUCTION: D should receive corrective help at his level of functioning in reading. Such instruction should stress word analysis skills, development of word meaning, and increasing of sight vocabulary. He should be provided with continuous opportunity to apply these skills in reading materials at about a third grade level.

In order for D to have some academic success, it will be necessary for his teachers to realize his severe learning disability and adjust their expectations accordingly. His disabilities are so severe that it will be almost impossible for him to grasp the content of the subject matter at his grade level.

SUMMARY

The above case reports serve to illustrate the fact that children with extreme reading problems do exist, whether we choose to call the problems dyslexia, or severe reading disability, or whatever. As a regular-school educator my concern is primarily what to do about them when they are identified.

The most extreme cases of dyslexia do not present an identification problem; educators and consultants agree on the diagnosis. At present dyslexic children are seldom offered an alternate curriculum, especially in the lower grades. There are attempts in some places to provide remediation through special support programs, but to my knowledge little proof of success exists to justify authorization of more than pilot studies at this time. I would welcome an alternate curriculum that would bypass rather than remediate while more research is carried out. Such a bookless curriculum is mentioned by Silverberg and Silverberg as a solution to the problems of dyslexic children. With all the modern technology available, it seems strange and unbelievable that we still offer primarily one single method of learning in our schools.

In the borderline cases the problem is more complex. Here the major problem for me is that if I choose to bypass intensive reading instruction, have I correctly classified the child, or have I set my expectations too low for that particular child? Would it not be kinder in the long run to follow the conservative outlook and *try* to teach all the children to read with all the power we have? What happens to the one who cannot learn when we are insensitive to his problem in our mass education system?

It seems to me that we in the regular school must stand ready to accept help from any quarter. We should cooperate with those seeking to study the problem whenever and wherever possible. We should enter into these studies with an open-minded attitude and a desire to learn. At the same time we must balance this posture with that imposed on us as public servants. We must be vigilant in protecting our clients from those who seek to profit by our confusion and caution at the expense of our clients.

We must proceed with caution—but we must not stagnate into inaction. This is a troubled position for the professional educator who seeks solutions to the problem. I believe that the problem can be solved only by joining with other disciplines in interdisciplinary groups. At present, although the problem cuts across disciplines, it is being handled in different ways by each. The most economical approach, therefore, seems to be one that would seek to find the successes in each discipline and integrate them into an effective program.

I would like to illustrate the problem in another way. The following remarks are taken from an actual report card that accompanied the records of a student in our center. I believe it serves to tell the story in yet another way and is a fitting summary of this chapter from the position of the regular-school practitioner.

GRADE CARD TEACHER COMMENTS FOR KEVIN

SCHOOL YEAR 1961-1962

First report: Kevin is working so hard and doing a good job. I'm not pushing him with his reading but letting him go as fast as he can. His work is much neater now than it was at the beginning of school.

Second report: Kevin is doing such a good job and trying so hard, I'm so proud of him. Thank you for helping him at home with his word cards and library books. I'm still letting him progress at his own rate in reading so that he feels secure. Maybe you could speak to him about keeping busy at his seat.

Third report: Kevin usually tries to do his best. He is especially trying to do neater work. He is well behaved in class, but sometimes is not so well behaved on the playground. He needs to read at home.

Final report (transfer information): I have certainly enjoyed Kevin. He has been well behaved on and off the playground. He is weak in reading but is progressing at his own pace. He always tries to do his best.

SCHOOL YEAR 1962-1963

First report: Kevin is such a sweet, helpful little boy. Always tries and certainly does his best. He just completed the first reader and made an average score. He started reading the second reader this week. Drill should be continued on vocabulary, as well as encouragement of library books. Kevin does well in numbers.

Second report: Kevin continues to work hard and certainly does his best. He needs constant drill on vocabulary and should be reading as much as possible at home. Good attitude—good work habits.

Third report: Kevin shows steady growth in all areas. He really tries and always wants to please. His reading is improving and he is doing very well in spelling and arithmetic.

Final report (transfer information): Kevin will continue work on level 6 in September. Kevin has certainly made a year's progress! I have enjoyed him in my class.

GRADE CARD TEACHER COMMENTS FOR KEVIN—cont'd

SCHOOL YEAR 1963-1964

First report: Kevin is a willing worker and he tries hard. At times he spends too much time talking.

Second report: Kevin has improved in written language. He still needs to spend less time talking in class. Often during the past two weeks Kevin has had to be reminded about obeying the playground rules.

Third report: Kevin has satisfactorily completed the second reader, book II, and is now reading in the third reader, book I. Kevin has made some improvement in his conduct.

Final report (transfer information): Kevin will be working in the fourth grade next fall.

SCHOOL YEAR 1964-1965

First report: Kevin is working hard to be a better student and to overcome his behavior difficulties.

Second report: Kevin's spelling has improved although not yet up to a B. He has worked in arithmetic but not consistently enough to keep up.

Third report: Kevin has made a real effort to improve in his studies this quarter.

Fourth report (final recommendations): Promoted to grade 5.

SCHOOL YEAR 1965-1966

No comments, assigned to grade 6.

SCHOOL YEAR 1966-1967

First report: Child is trying very hard. It is a slow and difficult process for Kevin, and I hope this report will not discourage him. He has *just found out* in the *last two weeks* how much he has to work, and he has made every effort to do so within the last few weeks. Give him a few words of encouragement. *Please.* I am sure he will continue to improve with encouragement.

Second report: Child has made a vast improvement but he still has a long way to go. Keep helping him, and give him a lot of encouragement and strict insistence on his doing his homework. He is on the right track. I just *hope* and pray he continues for his own sake. Thank you.

Third report: S— in science is for work Kevin did on the electric quiz board.

Fourth report: Good luck and God bless you. Kevin has made quite an achievement in this year but still has a long way to go. Please help him to understand that he *must* continue to go forward, and not backward. Assigned to grade 7.

REFERENCES

Bender, Lauretta: Use of the Visual-Motor Gestalt Test in the diagnosis of learning disabilities, J. Spec. Ed. 4:29, 1970.

Catterall, Calvin D.: Taxonomy of prescriptive interventions, J. Sch. Psychol. 8:5, 1970.

Edgerton, Roger B.: The cloak of competence, Berkeley, 1967, University of California Press.

Elam, Stanley: The age of accountability dawns in Texarkana, Phi Delta Kappan 51:509, 1970.

Environmental factors ruled out as a root of dyslexia symptoms, Pediatric News, Sept., 1968.

Goodman, Paul: High school is too much, Psychol. Today 4(5):25, 1970.

Henry, W. R.: Differential observation for visually related classroom problems, Symposium for Visual Perception, The Missouri Optometric Association, 1968.

Johnson, Mary: Programmed illiteracy in our schools, Winnipeg, 1970, Clarity.

Keeney, Arthur, and Keeney, Virginia T., editors: Dyslexia, St. Louis, 1968, The C. V. Mosby Co.

Oakland, Thomas: Diagnostic help 5¢: examiner is in, Psychol. Sch. 6:359, 1969.

The Philippines: the graduates, Newsweek **75**(**10**):38, 1970.

Rice, Donald: Learning disabilities: an investigation, J. Learn. Dis. 3:149, 193, 1970.

Rice, Ruth D.: Educo-therapy: a new approach to delinquent behavior, J. Learn. Dis. 3:16, 1970.

Silverberg, Norman E., Iversen, Iver A., and Silverberg, Margaret C.: A model for classifying children according to reading level, J. Learn. Dis. 2:634-643, 1969.

Silverberg, Norman E., and Silverberg, Margaret: The bookless curriculum: an educational alternative, J. Learn. Dis. 2:302-307, 1969.

Warner, L., et al.: Social class in America: a manual of procedure for the measurement of social status, New York, 1960, Harper & Row, Publishers.

Willson, Margaret: Clinical teaching and dyslexia, Read. Teach. **21**:730, 1968.

chapter 3

DIAGNOSIS AND TREATMENT OF THE DYSLEXIC CHILD

MARILYN McNAMEE LAMB AND PATRICIA TOOLEN

The purpose of this chapter is to help the reader identify the child of school age who has a learning disability as well as the preschool child with a potential learning disability. In addition, we would like to convey the idea that there is effective treatment available to such children. Six case histories that incorporate diagnostic and remedial procedures are presented.

The term "dyslexic" is used in the title as a catchall term. What we intend to discuss is the preschool or school-age child who is referred to the physician because of a failure to acquire skills commonly possessed by other children of the same chronological age. An eye examination reveals normal vision, or if a vision problem is found and corrected, the presenting problem still persists. Further investigation reveals normal hearing sensitivity and normal intelligence.

Few of these children are, or will be at school age, true "dyslexics." Many of them would be classified more accurately as children with some form of learning disability.

Among the many definitions of learning disability are the following two, which have been created by two of the leaders in the field of learning disabilities.

According to Kirk, "A learning disability refers to a retardation, disorder, or delayed development in one or more of the processes of speech, language, reading, spelling, writing, or arithmetic, resulting from possible cerebral dysfunction and/or emotional disturbance and not from mental retardation, sensory deprivation, or cultural or instructional factors."*

Bateman says, "Children who have learning disorders are those who manifest an educationally significant discrepance between their estimated intellectual potential and the actual level of performance related to basic disorders in the learning process, which may or may not be accompanied by demonstrable central nervous system dysfunction, and which are not secondary to generalized disturbance or sensory loss."†

---

*From Kirk, S. A.: Educating exceptional children, Boston, 1962, Houghton-Mifflin Co.
†From Bateman, B.: In Hellmuth, J., editor: Learning disorders, vol. 1, Seattle, 1965, Seattle Sequin School, p. 220.

Kirk's definition of learning disability implies an etiology of possible cerebral dysfunction and/or emotional disturbance and rules out mental retardation, whereas Bateman suggests that present measured intellectual function could be less than normal but excludes the presence of emotional disturbance as a possible cause. Many definitions of learning disability that have evolved since Kirk's and Bateman's would set down criteria for a learning disability that would include normal intelligence (at least for the school-age child) and would exclude emotional disturbance as a primary cause of the learning problem. Etiology would be considered unimportant, and behavior and learning style would be considered important.

In other words, then, the present concept of the learning-disabled child is that he is of normal intelligence, that he is peripherally intact, that he has been exposed to the appropriate learning experience, and that he is not culturally deprived or seriously emotionally disturbed. Despite all these strengths, he is not able to learn the things commonly learned by a child of his age who is of normal intelligence.

On more thorough examination he is found to have specific weaknesses in some areas necessary to learning by methods found to be successful with most children. This implies that he also has some areas of intact abilities, or strengths, that can be utilized in remediation of, or compensation for, his deficits.

It is important for the physician who has many child patients to be aware of the presence of learning disability and to be able to make a tentative diagnosis of the problem so that he can refer the child to the proper source for help.

Even more important than identification of the school-age child is the early identification of the preschool disabled learner. He is the child of 2½ or 3 years who has developed little or no language, has unintelligible speech, is physically immature, has poor coordination, is easily distracted, and/or exhibits hyperactivity or withdrawal symptoms. Early intervention is especially important because it can prevent the more complex and serious learning disability, and there is less chance of emotional complications.

TESTING THE DYSLEXIC CHILD

Some educated conjectures can be made as to who is the "learning-disabled child" by observing his behavior, listening to his speech and language, and taking a thorough case history. However, a test battery should be administered by a qualified psychologist to confirm this tentative diagnosis. It should include comprehensive tests of intellectual function, developmental diagnostic tests of achievement, and tests of visual and auditory perception, motor coordination, visual-perceptual-motor integration, and verbal expression.

The test battery should be flexible in regard to the age of the child and the kind of information sought. Some of the comprehensive instruments in popular use that have been found to be effective in diagnosis of learning disabilities are the Wechsler Intelligence Scale for Children (WISC), the Wechsler Preschool and

Primary Scale of Intelligence (WPPSI), and the Stanford-Binet Intelligence Scale (Terman and Merrill). For supportive information, the Bender Visual Motor Gestalt Test, the Beery Developmental Test of Visual-Motor Integration, the Goodenough Draw-A-Man Test, the Peabody Picture Vocabulary Test (PPVT) (Dunn), the Illinois Test of Psycholinguistic Abilities (ITPA) (McCarthy and Kirk), the Marianne Frostig Developmental Test of Visual Perception, the Metropolitan Achievement Tests (Durost et al.), and the Gates-McKillop Reading Diagnostic Tests can be used. There are many other adequate tools available. The above list is not meant to be comprehensive, by any means.

The tests themselves will not be described in detail. They are utilized to obtain scores but more importantly to sample behavior and to obtain a profile of developmental abilities. The tests measure the ability to abstract and conceptualize; the level of receptive and expressive vocabulary; the ability to receive, manipulate, and express ideas; short-term auditory and visual memory; grammar-syntax; the ability to deal with numbers; spatial orientation; visual and auditory discrimination; and the ability to synthesize, problem-solve, and form a gestalt from the given parts. The achievement tests measure past learning of formally taught materials that are considered important to school success. Scores on the achievement tests, in addition to reflecting the present level of academic function, can be used to predict success or failure at the next level.

The WISC and the WPPSI both yield a verbal IQ, a performance IQ, and a full-scale IQ. There are five or six verbal tests and five or six performance tests, all of which yield subtest scores from which a profile can be plotted. The WPPSI is suitable for children from the ages of 3 years 10 months through 6 years 6 months. The WISC is suitable for use with children from 5 years through 15 years 11 months of age.

The Stanford-Binet Intelligence Scale yields a mental age and an IQ. It can be used through the ages of 2 years through adulthood. Verbal and performance tests are interspersed throughout the test at each age level.

The Bender Visual Motor Gestalt Test and the Beery Developmental Test of Visual-Motor Integration are paper-pencil tests in which the child is asked to copy geometric designs. The Goodenough Draw-A-Man Test is another paper-pencil test that requires the child simply to draw a human figure. It yields both a mental age and an IQ. The Peabody Picture Vocabulary Test requires the child to identify one of four pictures on a page that matches the stimulus word presented aurally to the child. It too yields both a mental age and an IQ.

The ITPA is designed for use with children from 2 through 9½ years of age. It purports to test linguistic abilities in such a manner that a child's disability can be identified as a deficit in input, associative ability, or output in either the visual or the auditory channel. Remedial techniques that make use of the child's strengths and strengthen his weaknesses can then be used. There are twelve subtests, some of which tap abilities at the representational (meaningful) level, whereas others tap abilities at the automatic (nonmeaningful) level. Input, association, and output of both visual-perceptual-motor and auditory-vocal channels are tested at the representational level. At the automatic level, auditory and visual memory and closure, grammar-syntax, and sound-blending abilities are tested. The ITPA yields subtest scores for each ability, a total language age, and a total standard score.

The Marianne Frostig Developmental Test of Visual Perception consists of five subtests that measure perceptual skills. The subtests are called eye-motor co-ordination, figure-ground, form constancy, position in space, and spatial relations. Each subtest yields a scaled score and an age equivalent, and the total of the scaled scores yields a perceptual quotient. Frostig provides a planned sequence of activities that can be used in the remediation of perceptual deficits.

The Metropolitan Achievement Tests are organized on five levels. The child is tested on academic skills that have been formally taught and that must be mastered before he can succeed at the next level. Some diagnostic information can be gained from the test, but children with reading scores below expectancy level should be given an individual diagnostic test such as the Gates-McKillop Reading Diagnostic Test, which identifies specific areas of weakness in the reading skills.

OBSERVING ABNORMAL BEHAVIOR

Since the tests are utilized as behavior samples and to obtain profiles of development skills, it is important to observe and note behavior and test patterns that differ from normal. The normal child is goal oriented, he understands verbal directions appropriate for his age level, he is not unduly difficult to work with, he attends well, his speech and language are adequate for his age level, and his level of developmental skills is at least commensurate with his chronological age in all areas. His test profile would yield a nearly straight line at or above his age level. There would be little or no variability in performance either within or between subtests.

The mentally retarded child would also manifest little scatter within or among test scores. His profile of abilities would be fairly flat, with few peaks and valleys, but it would be consistently below his age level in all, or most, developmental skills. The retarded child may be hyperactive, may be poorly contained, may lose interest easily, and may be somewhat difficult to work with.

The learning-disabled child may exhibit some of the same types of behavior as the mentally retarded child. He may be withdrawn, hyperactive, poorly contained, or poorly motivated to perform, or he may exhibit none of these behavior patterns. He may perseverate in thought or action; he may have difficulty shifting from task to task; he may give inadequate responses initially, with adequate to superior responses coming later; he may need constant structuring and restructuring in order to stay with a task; he may have poor articulation and/or poor grammar-syntax for his age level; and he may manifest word-finding difficulty and problems with spatial orientation, number concepts, higher level abstraction, or paper-pencil tasks. He may need to have auditory stimuli repeated or rephrased, and he may be unable to block out extraneous auditory and/or visual stimuli. Despite all or some of these behavior patterns, however, he is still able to perform at a normal level on at least some tasks. His test pattern would show scatter within and/or between subtests, and his profile of abilities would be spiky, indicating strength in some areas and weakness in others.

CASE REPORTS

To illustrate how the diagnostic and remedial techniques are used, six case reports will be presented. Three of the children are of school age, and three are preschoolers. Only one of the children manifests symptoms that approximate a true "dyslexia" in the sense that he was totally unable to acquire the simplest sight words or even the names of the letters in the alphabet. Four are typical of the child who suffers from some degree of learning disability, and a case report of one retarded child is presented as a contrast to the others.

Case 1

This 7-year-old white male, one of twins, had an unremarkable prenatal and birth history. Postnatal history reveals that he was slow to walk (18 months of age) and was reportedly clumsy in gross motor activities. Language was delayed; he did not say simple words until the age of 2 years, after which time his articulation and language were poor. His twin's development was normal.

He had been referred first to an ophthalmologist and then to a neurologist by his public-school speech therapist because of his learning problem, his extremely poor articulation, and a transient nystagmus. Neurological findings were negative, vision was normal, and the child was referred to this speech and hearing clinic for further evaluation. The audiometric findings revealed normal hearing sensitivity but poor auditory discrimination. Speech and language evaluation indicated both poor articulation and poor language ability in relation to chronological age.

TESTING

BENDER GESTALT TEST. Psychometric evaluation revealed poor Bender gestalt reproductions for his age (Fig. 3-1), which would suggest a possible visual-perceptual-motor disability. His Goodenough IQ was 80, and the drawing (Fig. 3-2) was extremely immature. These scores further suggest the possibility of visual-perceptual-motor disability and/or poor development of body concept.

VERBAL TESTING. The PPVT IQ was 90, which suggests normal intellectual development in the area of understanding short, meaningful verbal stimuli. The WISC yielded a verbal IQ of 90, a performance IQ of 101, and a full-scale IQ of 95. These scores fall well within the normal range of intellectual function; yet this child was in danger of failing first grade. The difference between the verbal IQ of 90 and the performance IQ of 101 is clinically significant and suggestive of a possible language deficit. Inspection of the verbal subtest scaled scores reveals a range of 6 to 14. The normal range of subtest scores for a verbal IQ of 90 would be about 9 through 11. Performance scaled scores ranged from 10 to 11, which suggests fairly normal visual-perceptual-motor development. Actual behavior on the performance subtests, as well as intrasubtest scatter, suggests otherwise, however. He exhibited an inordinate amount of trial-and-error behavior before attaining correct solutions. Usually a child who can earn scores of 10 and 11 on the performance subtests executes the tests quickly and surely. His performance suggests, instead, a problem of integration and organization of the materials. He did have good autocritical ability and could recognize incorrect solutions and at least approximate better ones.

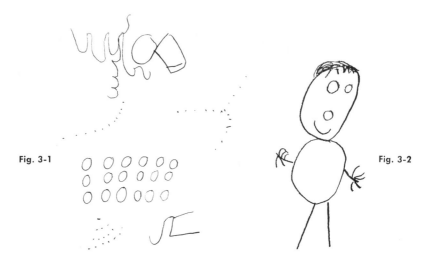

Fig. 3-1

Fig. 3-2

FIG. 3-1. Bender gestalt reproductions done by case 1, a 7-year-old white male with deficits in both language and visual-perceptual-motor skills. Drawings suggest immature visual-perceptual-motor skills.

FIG. 3-2. Goodenough man drawn by case 1, illustrating immature body concept for a child of his chronological age.

On the verbal tests, he manifested an inability to handle lengthy verbal messages. He often responded more adequately when the verbal stimuli were repeated or shortened. On abstract-conceptual tasks, his first responses were inadequate or at least quite concrete, but he was able to give very good abstract responses if given enough time to organize them. Language structure was quite poor for chronological age and level of intellectual function. Short-term auditory memory (for digits) was quite poor, and in addition he mixed the sequence of the digits in repetition. This poor ability for sequencing auditory vocal events in time was also reflected in his mixing sounds within words—for example, "aminals" for "animals" and "horse-riders-back" for "horseback riders." On the picture arrangement subtest, which is a performance subtest, he could sequence the story correctly but could not express the story verbally, which again suggests an expressive language deficit.

An ITPA was administered and pointed to the same findings. Subtest scores revealed low auditory-vocal abilities at both the representational and nonrepresentational levels. All visual-perceptual-motor abilities were at age level except for manual expression (gesturing). The responses on this task revealed poor fine motor coordination, confusion, and perseveration. He appeared to have difficulty orienting his movements in space and integrating and organizing motor movements.

On the auditory-vocal tasks, he again had difficulty with making verbal associations and abstractions, with verbal expression, and with short-term auditory memory, sound blending, and grammar-syntax. Although verbal deficit was his most overwhelming problem, he also manifested some disorganization of visual-perceptual-motor abilities.

ACHIEVEMENT TESTING. Achievement testing placed him about six months below grade level and one year below expectancy, based on chronological age and IQ. In summary, then, this child appeared to be a learning-disabled child, with his most serious deficits in the receptive, associative, and expressive aspects of language, and in the automatic functions necessary to facilitate these abilities. His reading deficit was primarily a result of poor ability to deal with verbal language. Two diagnostic-remedial sessions followed the psychological evaluation in order that recommendations could be made for follow-up by the classroom teacher and the speech clinician.

A structured situation was found to facilitate learning. Visual cues were found to be necessary for adequate verbal expression. The child was given further auditory cues through questions designed to help him reorganize his thoughts at a more abstract level. At the same time, auditory stimuli were shortened to the length that he could readily decode, and they were repeated or rephrased when necessary. New (less meaningful) stimuli coming in aurally needed several extra repetitions and, where possible, visual cues.

Some of the visual aids used were large action pictures to stimulate verbal expression. Appropriate questioning could elicit sentences correct in syntax, as well as generalizations, abstractions, new vocabulary words, and time sequence. Puzzles were used not only for eye-hand coordination and spatial organization but to elicit further verbal behavior. Tasks to improve sequencing in time, such as repeating a rhythm pattern, were used. Visual aids for auditory memory tasks—for example, remembering a sequence of colored sticks—were employed. Listening tasks and tasks from phonics workbooks were used to improve auditory discrimination. Parquetry blocks were used as visual cues for directions given aurally.

This child always improved his responses when given a few warm-up trials and when given extra time and cues to organize a better response. He often needed to actually produce his verbal response and to think about it again before he could give a verbal response at a higher level.

This boy was referred to the clinic for diagnosis only and therefore was not placed in therapy other than the two diagnostic sessions. A complete report, which stressed the idea that verbal language skills must precede reading skills, was sent to both the classroom teacher and the speech clinician. Both reported good success in working with the child and felt that the findings had helped them in understanding him better and in knowing how to work with him.

Case 2

This white female, age 11½ years, was referred to the clinic because of poor articulation and nonfluent verbal behavior. The family history revealed poor articulation and stuttering in other family members. Prenatal and birth histories were negative. Early motor development was normal, but toilet training and acquisition of language were delayed. This child was hyperactive and began to have petit mal seizures at the age of 4 years. She was placed on medications for seizures and hyperactivity until 9 years of age, when EEG tracings were found to be normal. Medication for the seizures was terminated at that time, with no recurrence of the seizures. Medication for hyperactivity was continued.

Although the initial referral was for stuttering and poor articulation, routine evaluation brought to light a language deficit and mild visual-perceptual-motor involvement, as well as academic retardation. Hearing evaluation revealed normal hearing sensitivity but poor auditory discrimination.

TESTING

BENDER GESTALT TEST. The Bender gestalt test and the Goodenough Draw-A-Man Test suggested immaturity, if not possible organic involvement. Verbal receptive IQ (PPVT) was 93, and the WISC full-scale IQ was 99 (verbal IQ, 92; performance IQ, 107). This difference between verbal and performance scores is quite significant clinically and suggests a depression of overall language ability in relation to performance abilities. Performance subtest scores were all within normal range, whereas verbal subtest scores manifested a good deal of both intratest and intertest variability. The range of verbal scores was from 7 to 11. The ITPA showed deficits in grammar-syntax and short-term auditory memory in the auditory-vocal channel, and a deficit in motor encoding in the visual-motor channel.

Test behavior revealed good articulation skills in isolated words, but speech rapidly became unintelligible in conversation. In addition to her stuttering, spontaneous conversational speech was characterized by substitutions, mixing of the order, and the addition or omission of sounds within a word—for example, "whiksers" for "whiskers," "Columbius" for "Columbus," and "magify" for "magnify." Word-finding difficulties were obvious. She called a "Band-Aid" a "first-aid" and a "hinge" a "notch." Responses that should have been organized and abstract were disorganized and rambling. Language structure, which should be an automatic activity for a child of this age, was quite poor; for example, she would say: "them am both . . . ," and "them am both am . . . ." She had a rather short attention span but was able to improve her performance with external structure.

READING TEST. The Gates-McKillop Reading Diagnostic Tests indicated a reading level of third grade, sixth month, which for her indicated an academic retardation of at least three years. She had difficulty with word gestalts. Phonetically, she could attack one-syllable words, but on two-syllable words, the first would be correct and the second incorrect. This appeared to be caused by her lack of knowledge of word meanings. This girl appeared to have acquired the basic mechanical reading skills but was poor on tasks requiring good sentence sense, good vocabulary, organization, speed, and comprehension, which also suggests a deficit in higher-level language function rather than a problem with the mechanics of reading. She was also lacking in self-confidence. This child, again, would be diagnosed as having a learning disability, with deficits in language skills.

THERAPY

Remediation included instruction and practice in the following areas:
1. Structured language tasks making use of clear-cut verbal goals and short responses
2. Auditory discrimination tasks and tasks to teach sequencing of auditory events in time
3. The use of visual aids to elicit shorter but syntactically correct responses, to build concepts, and to increase vocabulary
4. Practice in structured verbal expression, retelling short stories, completing analogies, categorizing, and learning new vocabulary (she was not allowed to ramble when giving verbal responses)

Stuttering therapy was not used, since it was felt that the cause of the nonfluent behavior and poor reading was the child's poor automatic ability for grammar-syntax and her inability to organize verbal responses, as well as her poor grasp of language generally.

Improvement was noted in both expressive language and reading for meaning within six weeks. In addition, the stuttering behavior diminished.

Case 3

This white male, 8 years 8 months of age, was referred to the clinic by an ophthalmologist because of dyslexia. This child manifested the most severe reading disability seen in the combined twenty-year clinical experience of the authors.

This child had been evaluated by other agencies at the age of 6 years and again at the age of 7 years because of an inability to learn to read. There was a history of dyslexia in the family. Two older brothers, now in their teens, had been diagnosed as dyslexic. One of the brothers has seizures, and the other a history of hyperactivity. The patient himself had a negative prenatal and birth history. Early development in both language and motor skills was normal. His mother felt that he was an active child but would not have called him hyperactive. He had been retained twice in first grade, had had summer tutoring, and was in second grade and still not reading at even the preprimer level at the time of the evaluation.

Reading-readiness ability was superior as measured by the Metropolitan Readiness Tests, but he could not begin to attack the reading tasks at the next level. He was, at the age of 8 years 8 months, still hyperactive. He had been on medication for hyperactivity as a younger child, although the mother reported that medication did not help. Vision was normal. Audiometric evaluation revealed normal hearing sensitivity. Auditory discrimination was found to be poor during the diagnostic therapy sessions. Articulation, language structure, and general level of language was adequate. Reports from other agencies, however, suggested that there had been some immaturity in both speech and language when the child was younger, and more hyperactive behavior than his mother likes to admit.

Behavior presently appeared to be a problem because of his hyperactivity and impulsivity. The boy seemed to be in tremendous need of external structure. His inner controls were quite poor. For example, the evaluation took three sessions, and during one particularly long session, he was unable to tolerate staying at the worktable. He crawled under the table, moved to a smaller chair across the room, and rolled on the floor, in addition to becoming out of control verbally. He was quite difficult to work with because of his short attention span and his inability to concentrate on the task at hand. Neither mother nor school admitted any behavior difficulties, however.

TESTING

Overall intellectual function fell well within normal limits. Receptive verbal IQ, as measured on the PPVT, was 119, which is at the high end of the bright-normal continuum, bordering on superior. Understanding of verbal concepts presented aurally with visual cues was quite good.

Verbal IQ on the WISC was 100, performance IQ was 97, and full-scale IQ was 99, which is normal. There was a good deal of both intertest and intratest variability. The range in both verbal and performance subtest scores was from 8 to 12. Ability for nonschool incidental learning was superior. Commonsense items were completed fairly well. The arithmetic score was poor but was thought to be a reflection of his impulsivity and disinhibition rather than a reflection of poor number concepts per se. Vocabulary (verbal concepts) and similarities (abstractions) subtest scores were normal to superior; however, examination of the quality of the responses revealed many concrete (1 point) responses. This type of response indicates inability for higher level conceptualization and abstraction. Short-term auditory memory for nonmeaningful materials (digit span) was poor. Verbal responses were given in a rambling style almost as if he were free-associating. He needed external control from the examiner to keep his responses relevant. Initially, responses were often impulsive and illogical but became more adequate when he was given external structure by the examiner.

Inadequacy was also noted on some visual-perceptual-motor tasks. The Bender gestalt designs (Fig. 3-3) were poorly executed for a boy of his age. His Goodenough drawing (Fig. 3-4) revealed a poor concept of body image. He had an extremely poor ability to distinguish essentials from nonessentials, and he responded impulsively. His ability to sequence a series of pictures into a sensible story and to verbalize the story was superior. However, he did not have a firmly established habit of proceeding from left to right, which is a learned skill and

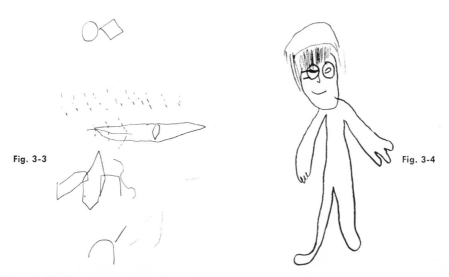

Fig. 3-3   Fig. 3-4

FIG. 3-3. Bender gestalt reproductions done by case 3, an 8-year 8-month-old while male referred for dyslexia. Drawings reflect impulsivity.
FIG. 3-4. Goodenough man drawn by case 3, reflecting impulsivity and inadequate body image.

essential to good reading. The ability to synthesize and abstract principles nonverbally was excellent, although organization depending on visual-spatial cues was poor. He appeared to have difficulty with new nonmeaningful visual learning and with visual memory of nonmeaningful materials.

He appeared, then, to be receiving meaningful, auditory stimuli adequately, although he handled nonmeaningful materials poorly. He was deficient in his ability to organize and express meaningful verbal communication. He appeared to have some initial confusion organizing meaningful visual stimuli but was able to succeed if given extra structure. Language structure (grammar-syntax) was adequate, as was vocabulary.

Test scores alone did not adequately reflect the severity of this child's disability. Although he had deficits in auditory and visual memory, auditory perception, higher-level language function, and verbal expression, scores were no poorer than those of many other learning-disabled children. Yet in reading he had made no measurable progress after three years in school. What the test scores did not reflect was the behavior of this child in attaining his test scores. His most outstanding deficit seemed to be his inability to organize and control his own behavior and to structure tasks for himself so as to derive meaning from them.

Recommendations for this child were as follows:

1. A structured situation to help reduce irrelevant stimuli and to help him discriminate the relevant aspects of the task; use of aids which would facilitate organization for him
2. Practice in auditory discrimination, auditory closure, and sound blending
3. Practice in abstracting, generalizing, categorizing, and solving analogies
4. Structure of verbal output to discourage irrelevant responses
5. Practice in visual sequencing from left to right
6. Presentation of meaningful wholes when possible, rather than nonmeaningful parts

THERAPY

After the psychometric evaluation, reading therapy was initiated by the educational therapist. Initially during the sessions there was little distractibility and hyperactivity. However, as time progressed, this behavior became more and more frequent. At this time the psychologist and therapist recommended that the child again be put on medication. Medication did seem to lessen his distractibility and hyperactivity, and the attention span was increased.

Since he had been unable to learn his alphabet or any sight words after three years in school, it was thought that a method utilizing a kinesthetic approach to the whole word rather than a phonetic approach should be used. The Fernald method (Fernald and Keller) was decided on. In addition, sounds of the alphabet letters, but not letter names, were practiced, and practice in structuring verbal expression was given.

This child's biggest interest was fishing. Some discussion on the topic preceded the learning of individual words. The following are the words he wanted to know: salmon, bass, cod, fish, catfish, bait, reel, tackle, and rod. Three words were learned the first day and two words during the second lesson. Because the child developed some disinterest in learning only single words, a few helping words were taught so that he could make some original sentences. The words were put on individual cards for motivational purposes. Examples of the sentences are as follows:

1. I can fish.
2. I can go fishing.
3. Three of us are going fishing.

After the sentences, the next step was to make his own "story" in booklet form. The completed book is shown in Fig. 3-5. Words that made up the sentences were color cued. Those in blue (not underlined) were the ones he had learned from the Fernald method, and those in red (underlined) were simple sight words learned at school or in therapy. Many of the sight words were remembered because of context clues or picture clues.

Therapy was terminated at the end of the school year, and the child was enrolled in a summer tutoring program at his own school.

The following are the recommendations made for his summer program:

1. Continued work with the sounds (not the letter names) of the alphabet

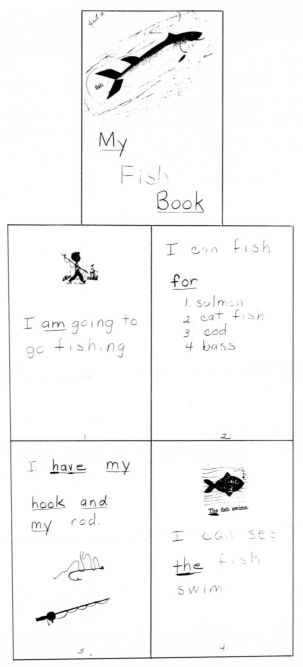

FIG. 3-5. The completed book done by case 3, illustrating use of words the child wanted to learn, in a context meaningful to him.

2. Phonics worksheets for practice on beginning sounds (used to familiarize the child with the configuration of the letters; only the sounds should be taught)
3. Fernald method to be continued; sequence of introducing words should be followed very carefully
4. Introduction of configurations of words to give the child practice in seeing the whole words; for example, salmon, rod, or fish
5. Practice on visual and auditory memory activities and auditory discrimination tasks
    a. Series of cubed blocks or shapes (the child looks at them; the therapist then mixes them up so that the child may fix them in the correct sequence, working from left to right)
    b. Picture cards or other materials (substituted for the blocks)
    c. Memory activities, in which similar words or digits are given and then repeated
    d. For auditory discrimination, a set of three words—two rhyming words and one that does not rhyme (the child identifies the two rhyming words or the word which does not rhyme)
6. Structured situation in which to work

At the end of the summer a follow-up report from the school stated that the Fernald method was the only method by which he had been able to learn. Sixty-eight new words were learned during the summer. Some improvement was shown in consonant sounds, reading vocabulary, word meanings, reading games, and listening.

Case 4

This white female with Treacher-Collins syndrome was seen for psychometrics at the clinic at the age of 3 years. She initially came to the clinic at 2 years 6 months of age because she had not acquired any expressive language. The history revealed that she had always been below age level in visual-perceptual-motor skills as well as in language development. Her behavior was characterized by drooling, immaturity, and flat affect; however, she was responsive to commands. She had a fluctuating bilateral conductive hearing loss.

Testing

Psychometric testing measured a relatively low verbal-receptive IQ (73) as seen on the PPVT. In Fig. 3-6 her Goodenough drawing shows as scribbles only. Her Beery reproductions were also scribbles only. By the age of 3 years a child should be able to reproduce a circle. Stanford-Binet IQ was 82, which placed her at the lower end of the dull-normal range and close to the range of borderline mental retardation. A definite unevenness in development was revealed by the spread of successes and failures. No basal age was established, which means that she had not yet mastered some tasks at the year II level; yet she did pass other tasks at

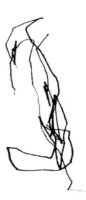

Fig. 3-6. Goodenough man drawn by case 4, a 3-year-old white female with Treacher-Collins syndrome. The drawing illustrates immature visual-perceptual–motor skills and body image for a child of her age.

the year III-6 level. The tasks failed at the year II and year II-6 levels were those which required verbal responses. She was able to succeed on both verbal-receptive tasks and visual-perceptual-motor tasks at the year II level. At year III and III-6 she succeeded only in visual-memory and visual discrimination tasks.

Although this child's overall IQ fell at the low end of the dull-normal range, she had acquired some skills at or even above her age level. This finding suggests good potential for further intellectual growth. Specific weaknesses seemed to be in the areas of short-term auditory memory, verbal expression, and fine motor coordination. Visual discrimination, visual memory, and auditory decoding of meaningful verbal stimuli appeared adequate. However, she required that meaningful verbal stimuli be embedded in either a visual or a verbal contextual situation.

The mother was counseled as to the present intellectual status of her child and her prognosis for good progress.

LANGUAGE THERAPY

The first four months of therapy consisted of monthly language therapy sessions which the mother observed in order to be able to continue the activities at home. At the time of the psychometric evaluation it was decided that this child would profit from twice-weekly language therapy sessions in which short verbal stimuli were presented and short verbal responses were encouraged. After three months of individual language therapy it was felt that she was mature enough for a language class with three or four other children of her age.

The other children in the language class knew some single words and a few phrases. As this child began to socialize with the others and participate in game activities, she began to say a few single words, such as "home," "da," and "up." More words were introduced by presenting actual objects and pictures in categories. Blocks, puzzles, and other toys were utilized to establish prenursery skills. The language class was terminated after eight months, at which time she had a fairly good vocabulary of single words.

This child was then seen in individual therapy and at the same time was enrolled in nursery school. The individual therapy began with the introduction of two-word phrases. At the beginning a verb-noun combination—for example, "eat pie" and "ride bike"—was used. As time progressed, a short sentence using a noun, such as "girl," "boy," "da," "mom," or the pronoun "I," with a verb and noun was introduced.

Before psychometric retesting was scheduled the following basic skills were mastered:

1. In visual-perceptual development, this child was capable of putting together simple three- and four-piece puzzles. The vertical and horizontal lines and the square were copied correctly on the pegboard. The lines were drawn correctly. The square was drawn, although somewhat crudely. Reproductions of simple block designs and simple tasks involving size, color, and form discrimination were accomplished with difficulty only in the fine motor area.

2. Some progress was made in both gross and fine motor areas, but this child still seemed to exhibit difficulty with some tasks—for example, hopping on one foot—in the gross motor area and paper-and-pencil tasks in the fine motor area.

3. In the receptive language area, she no longer appeared to be delayed in her development. She was able to identify pictures from verbal stimuli and to follow directions.

Much progress was made in the area of expressive language. She began with single words, then phrases, and at this time used simple sentences, although in spontaneous speech she might still use only phrases. Articles were still lacking from her vocabulary, but she understood and used the following prepositions: "in," "on," and "under." Categorization of pictures and objects was accomplished. Colors and numbers up to six were learned.

This child was reevaluated at 5 years 3 months of age—two years and three months after the initial evaluation. She had been in therapy for approximately two and one-half years. Both mother and therapist were pleased with the growth in language and motor skills.

THERAPY EVALUATION

Test results at the time of the reevaluation indicated a 20-point jump in verbal receptive ability (from a PPVT IQ of 73 to a PPVT IQ of 94), which reflected growth in understanding verbal concepts as well as increased ability to deal with meaningful stimuli out of context.

Her Goodenough man, as seen in Fig. 3-7, showed a mental age of 4 years 6 months and an IQ of 86. Body image was still quite poor, but she was able to conceptualize some body parts, including eyebrows, which is a rather mature concept for a child of her age.

The Stanford-Binet IQ jumped from 82, low dull-normal, to 95, mid-normal, which was fairly dramatic. She now had solidly acquired skills up to the year IV level. Development of skills was uneven from the IV to VII year levels. Again, she failed some items below her age level and passed some above her age level, which indicates not only that some unevenness of development was still present but that there will probably still be more intellectual growth. She still switched hands at the midline if the situation was unstructured, which indicates a poorly organized body concept. Short-term auditory memory was still poor in relation to chronological age, and she had inordinate difficulty sequencing auditory input. She also fell below her age level in some visual-perceptual-motor tasks. She could define vocabulary words at her age level and used spontaneous language in conversation. Language structure was still poor for her age level. Even though overall IQ was normal, then, this child was still probably going to have learning problems.

Recommendations were to continue language therapy, tying in the visual-perceptual-motor skills, and to continue preschool another year rather than to enter kindergarten.

At this time specific recommendations included beginning work in generalizing and abstracting, and continuation of building language structure, number concepts, and categorization. Activities in the visual-perceptual-motor area included tracing, use of templates and puzzles, and block building to help with spatial orientation. Left-right sequencing activities, folding, cutting, and reproducing bead and block patterns should be included in her activities. Building of gross motor skills would include swimming, using a swing set, walking board, tricycle, and jumping rope.

It is difficult to say that early identification and remediation was the sole cause of increased verbal, motor, and social skills, since she may well have developed these skills to at least some extent with no intervention. It is unlikely, however, that a child with such poor abilities,

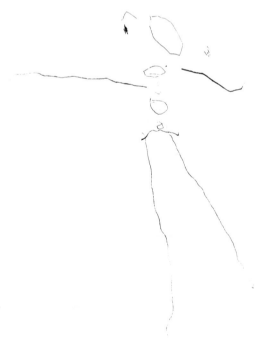

FIG. 3-7. Goodenough man drawn by the same child at the age of 5 years 3 months. The drawing suggests that this child still has immature fine motor skills and body concept for her age.

lack of curiosity, and goal direction would accomplish these tasks spontaneously to the level attained in her two and one-half years of therapy.

This child still has deficits that may cause her to be classified as a learning-disabled child throughout her early school years; however, she will probably enter school with a higher level of readiness than she would have without therapy. Further, areas of strength and weakness have been identified and a program of effective remedial techniques has been established for use by her preschool teacher. A child like this should be reevaluated, then, before she enters first grade in order to measure progress and to help determine whether she will be able to succeed at the first grade level in a regular class with no extra help, whether she will be able to succeed in a first grade class with extra help in specific skills, or whether she should be placed in a class for learning-disabled children.

Case 5

A white female, 3 years 9 months of age, was referred to the clinic by her pediatrician because of a failure to develop language skills. Prenatal and birth histories were negative. In addition to poor language development there was some delay in acquisition of motor skills. At the age of 3 years she had had an operation to correct strabismus and was now wearing glasses. Audiometric examination revealed essentially normal hearing sensitivity. Auditory discrimination could not be tested because she had only one "word" in her repertoire of expressive language. The "word" was "aguk," which is interesting because it contains two syllables and some sounds that are somewhat advanced developmentally. This suggests that she was capable of producing the sounds necessary for words and that if she could be given some names for things, she would be able to articulate them well. She was interested in imitating sounds made by the examiner and was able to do so, and she was even able to approximate some simple words.

Testing

Psychometric test results include a PPVT IQ of 76, which, although suggestive of borderline mental retardation, indicates a verbal receptive ability much superior to her expressive language skills. The Goodenough man (Fig. 3-8) was only a scribble, which suggests a developmental level of 2 to 2½ years. The scribble was controlled and circular, which indicates some beginning of autocritical ability and beginning motor control.

The Stanford-Binet IQ was 64 and the mental age was 2 years 5 months. This score falls well within the range of mental retardation.

With a chronological age of 3 years 9 months, this child had not yet developed the expressive language skills necessary to succeed at the year II level of the Stanford-Binet scale. On the positive side, she found the performance tasks at the year II and year II-6 levels quite

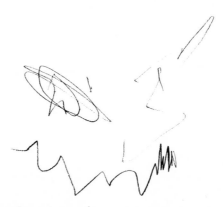

Fig. 3-8. Goodenough man drawn by case 5, a 3-year 9-month white female who has no expressive language. The drawing is below age level.

easy and was able to succeed on most of the year III tasks with difficulty. She then was able to succeed on visual discrimination tasks and verbal reception tasks at her age level.

Clearly, then, this child appeared to have attained some skills appropriate to her age level, which was contraindicative of mental retardation even though her total IQ scores fell within the range of mental retardation.

The child's mother was counseled as to the present level of intellectual function as well as the prognosis of potentially better function. Individual language therapy with eventual placement in a small group was begun.

THERAPY

Group placement appeared to stimulate the acquisition of expressive language for this child. She enjoyed the group activities and participated very well. It was through activities, such as naming pieces of play furniture and playing color word games, that she began to use single words. As the children took turns at naming pieces of furniture or clothing, this little girl took her turn because she was part of the group. As she had practice over a period of time in this setting, it was apparent that she was building a good single-word vocabulary. The parents were informed of the words learned after the sessions, and they stimulated production of these words at home.

Words that are useful in a child's everyday life were taught in categories, as were words of particular interest to the child. In this child's case the subject of interest was a dog. She wanted a dog very much and learned how to express this want verbally, as well as learning words used to describe a dog, such as "big," "black," "bow-wow."

At the termination of the language class, this child had 30 single words, both nouns and verbs, in her expressive vocabulary.

As individual therapy continued, the child was able to join a verb and a noun by using a picture cue, and to describe an action she herself performed. Articles were lacking from her vocabulary, although she did understand and begin to use prepositions such as "in," "on," and "under." Phrases and simple sentences were acquired, although in automatic speech she often used only phrases.

It is interesting to note that this child had a younger brother who was not talking. As this patient progressed in language development, the mother reported that the younger brother also showed much improvement. When the little brother visited the clinic with his sister at a later time, it was observed that his expressive language was normal for his age level.

Progress was made in the gross and fine motor areas, although she still exhibited difficulty with tasks expected at her age level—for example, hopping on one foot in the gross motor area, and working with paper and pencil in the fine motor area.

In visual-perception development the following tasks were accomplished:
1. Simple three- and four-piece puzzles
2. Simple tasks involving size, color, and form discrimination
3. Sequencing of beads on a string
4. Arrangement of vertical and horizontal lines, a square, and an X on a pegboard (she still exhibited a difficult time in drawing the square and X, although she always attempted the drawing)

THERAPY EVALUATION

This little girl was reevaluated at the age of 4 years 4 months of age after seven months of therapy. Behavior was generally more mature than before, and she appeared more self-confident. She had by now acquired some expressive language, and articulation was good.

PPVT IQ was now 101 (normal), which is an increase of 25 points and reflects a dramatic growth in understanding verbal concepts. Her Stanford-Binet IQ had jumped from 64 (mentally defective) to 97 (normal). She was now able to succeed on all verbal-expressive tasks at the II-6 level, and she approached success on many of the verbal-expressive tasks at the year III level. She still showed a deficit in short-term auditory memory, naming objects from pictures, language structure and organization, and expression of adequate verbal responses.

Thus, even though intellectual function was measured as being within the normal range,

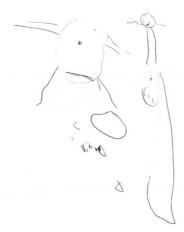

FIG. 3-9. Goodenough man drawn by case 5 at the age of 5 years 4 months. The drawing is adequate at the 4-year 6-month level; and perseveration is noted.

she still showed a spread of successes and failures from the three- to six-year level. At this time individual language therapy was continued and she was enrolled in a regular preschool program.

Reevaluation one year later at the age of 5 years 4 months yielded a Stanford-Binet IQ that had stabilized in the mid-90 range, with the scatter reduced. She has now filled in some gaps at the lower levels of language development. Her Goodenough man (Fig. 3-9) now shows development of body concepts at the IV-6 level.

Language structure and short-term auditory memory are still poor, but she can now define vocabulary words at the year V level, and she can organize fairly good verbal responses. Motor skills at the year V level are weak.

During the course of therapy the family bought a new home in a remote rural area where there are no special education facilities or adequate nursery schools. Therefore, the recommendation made to the mother at this time was to place the child in kindergarten, with the idea that she may spend two years at that level. Had the family remained in the local area, the recommendation would have been another year of preschool and, at age 6 years, evaluation for possible placement in a special education class for learning-disabled children of normal intelligence.

Psychological and educational test results and recommendations were sent to the child's school, along with progress reports from the therapist.

The kindergarten teacher, then, would have an understanding of the child and some idea of where to begin working with her, what techniques have been successful, and what skills she must emphasize.

Case 6

This case is presented as a contrast to the other five cases. The child was referred to the clinic by her pediatrician because of poor articulation skills at the age of 4 years. Prenatal and birth history were negative. Early development was slow in all areas.

Test results at the age of 4 years yielded a WPPSI IQ of 63. The verbal IQ of 79 and performance IQ of 53 indicate a sizable difference between language and visual-perceptual-motor skills; however, even her best abilities were considerably below her age level, and all IQ scores fell within the range of mental retardation. There was no intertest or intratest scatter.

Language structure and verbal expression were below her age level, and articulation was extremely poor. Speech therapy was initated because of the severity of the articulation problem. Progress was slow but steady. When articulation skills were improved enough for her to be intelligible, therapy plans were altered to include work in language and visual-perceptual-motor skills. The mother was counseled as to the child's present intellectual function and was introduced to the idea that she would probably need special education at school age. Since this child was hyperactive and distractible, it was further recommended that the parents consult their physician, with the idea of placing the child on medication. This recommendation was carried out; the hyperactivity was noticeably reduced, and the ability to attend and the level of tolerance for frustration were increased.

Because it was felt that at the age of 5 years she would not be ready to cope with kindergarten-level tasks, she was enrolled in a preschool program. At the age of 6 years she was enrolled in kindergarten in the mornings and participated in a small-group situation at the clinic two afternoons per week.

TESTING

An ITPA was administered before she was placed in the small-group situation at the age of 6 years. The test pattern revealed a flat profile, with all skills below her age level with the exception of sound blending, which was felt to be inflated by the extensive speech therapy. There was also an extreme dip in auditory association, which taps a higher level of abstracting ability and is highly correlated with IQ measurements. No specific recommendations for remediation were made for therapy from psychometric testing at this time, since the child was low in all abilities.

Retesting with the ITPA six months later revealed no important changes in her pattern of skills. Development was still fairly even across skills, with the results of all subtests significantly below her age level. Visual reception and auditory association improved, probably because of specific teaching of these skills by the therapist. In the meantime, without the coaching of the speech therapist, some ability to blend sounds was lost.

A readministration of the WPPSI during the same month revealed a full-scale IQ of 66, a verbal IQ of 75, and a performance IQ of 62. The gap between verbal and performance abilities was closing, but the full-scale IQ remained stable within the range of the educable mentally retarded. There was, as before, no intratest or intertest scatter.

Even though this child received more than two years of almost individualized therapy in language and visual-perceptual-motor development, she showed only maintenance of her rate of intellectual growth and no growth in the rate of development. This child coped with the prereadiness and readiness skills presented to her; however, the time involved and the repetition necessary for learning the skills far exceeded that which was required for the other children.

THERAPY RESULTS

At the age of 7 years she was enrolled in first grade and was able to compete successfully in the slowest reading group; by the end of the year she had mastered what would be considered one semester's work in reading. At this time a decision was made to refer her to special education services for an evaluation and possible class placement in a class for educable mentally retarded children. She did benefit from therapy to the extent that she was able to maintain newly learned skills and thereby avoid failure in kindergarten and first grade. The mother learned techniques for management of behavior and follow-up on specific skills taught during therapy sessions. She also came to be able to accept the idea that her child was going to need special education.

The basic difference between this child and the others was that there was little variability within or between subtests, that none of the abilities measured reached her age level, and that reevaluation showed no increase in the rate of intellectual development. Her pattern of skills was flat and significantly below the norms for her age group, and remained stable over a period of time even with intensive stimulation.

SUMMARY

The six case reports presented were chosen because the children in the reports typify the kind of child referred for psychoeducational evaluation and therapy.

Five of the six were learning-disabled children. All six were subsequently placed in developmental or remedial educational therapy.

Clinically, the learning-disabled children present a picture of slow acquisition of at least one important developmental skill. They may also exhibit some deviant behavior patterns such as hyperactivity, withdrawal, acting out, or destructiveness. The behavior disorders so often seen along with learning disorders occur because the child may not be able to understand verbal commands, he may be frustrated by his inability to express himself verbally, he may not have the internal language necessary for good inner control, or he may be a "driven" child.

These behavior patterns, in addition to being harmful in themselves, result in poor interpersonal relationships. Parents often do not know how to control the behavior and react ineffectively or punitively. They begin to feel they are failures as parents and that working with the child is a hopeless task.

The older child may no longer show the gross signs of poor articulation, lack of language development, extreme hyperactivity, and clumsiness. His receptive and expressive language may appear adequate in casual conversation. His presenting complaint may be simply that he is not achieving in school. He may, by now, be a disappointment to his parents because of disobedience, "laziness," school falure, and/or failure in interpersonal relationships.

The standardized testing situation ordinarily will not reveal this kind of poor behavior because it is a highly structured situation and takes place in an unstimulating environment. Further, the tests are designed to begin at a 100% success level, which almost assures cooperation. Sometimes poor behavior will begin to manifest itself when the level of difficulty of the tasks become frustrating, when testing time has been too long, if interruptions occur, or if the examiner presents tasks that are free and unstructured.

The parent often expresses amazement at the child's cooperation. This can be a good opportunity to help the parent see that the child can be cooperative and to point out to him the elements in the situation which helped the child to function well.

The standardized testing situation will, however, give the child the opportunity to exhibit his strengths and weaknesses in intellectual functioning. The learning-disabled child will manifest at least some, and perhaps many, of the following behavior patterns: difficulty in attending, poor auditory and/or visual discrimination, poor auditory and/or visual memory for nonmeaningful material, poor articulation, poor language structure, inability to decode meaningful auditory or visual stimuli, inability to organize and structure ideas presented aurally and/or visually, inability to express these ideas verbally or motorically, inability to distinguish between the relevant and the irrelevant, and inability to tune out extraneous stimuli. He may be unable to abstract and conceptualize, visual perception may be poor, vocabulary may be inadequate, and motor skills may be deficient.

The test protocol of a learning-disabled child will manifest a pattern of inconsistent responding within subtest areas and/or between subtest areas. If drawn on a graph, the pattern would be one of peaks and valleys instead of the almost straight line which the normal child produces. A retarded child, on the other hand, will also produce an almost straight line if his abilities are graphed, but the line will be significantly below the line representing the abilities of the normal child.

The educational therapist will begin her therapy with the information gained through the psychological evaluation. She may first make an educational evaluation, especially with a school-age child. She will want to find out how much academic retardation is actually present and what specific areas of reading, if he is reading, the child cannot cope with. He may have difficulty discriminating one sound from another or one letter from another, he may have poor auditory memory for sounds or poor visual memory for letters or words, or he may be unable to associate the phoneme (sound) with the grapheme (the letters that visually symbolize the sound). He may be able to read words very well, but be unable to comprehend the sentences or paragraphs he has read because of poor language function.

The therapist begins work with the child knowing his intellectual and academic strengths and weaknesses. She now has some immediate goals for therapy. Because she knows the level at which the child is presently working in the particular skill she wants to improve, she can set up a situation in which the child will meet with success 90% of the time. She employs a working knowledge of child development, learning theory, and behavior modification techniques.

The therapist may have to structure the environment to be free of extraneous auditory and/or visual stimuli. She may have to structure the environment to help the child "make sense" of it. She may have to give him several "warm up" trials each time she switches tasks. She may use visual stimuli to elicit the desired language behavior or verbal cues to structure visual-perceptual-motor tasks. Careful attention must be given to time limits and frustration level so that tasks are stopped while the child is still working at a high rate of success.

In addition to remediation of specific deficits, there are three long-term goals for educational therapy. The first goal is to teach the child to learn independently by teaching him to cope with his environment. One child may be taught that he must have many repetitions of any new material reaching him aurally or visually. He might be taught to associate a visual cue with an auditory stimulus. He may need to learn to segment long assignments into small sections, with a rest between sections. He may need to learn that he will work best in a quiet and austere room rather than in the middle of the family room. Another child may have to learn to outline all his work, to make a list of things to be done in their proper order, to underline in heavy ink, or to spell kinesthetically.

The second long-term goal of the educational therapist is to improve the child's self-concept. This is one purpose of the use of the 90% success situation. Often the educational therapy sessions are the first success situations the child has experienced. He begins to see that he can succeed and that he can learn. One success prepares the way for another. With successful experience the self-concept changes from one of unworthiness and helplessness to one of worthwhileness and self-direction. The feeling of achievement becomes a reward for the task accomplished as well as motivation to begin the next task. An internal sense of structure and self-direction begins to replace the need for external structure and reward.

The third goal of educational therapy is to help the parent learn how to teach his child effectively. The involvement of the parent begins with the initial interpretation of test results and recommendations. The parent often leaves the initial interview quite relieved that, not only is there an explanation for the child's behavior, but there are some things that can be done to help him. He also often loses his sense of guilt over both the child's behavior and his own ineffectiveness in dealing with him.

The parent is allowed to observe therapy sessions and has frequent conferences with the therapist. Through observation of techniques and conferences with the therapist, the parent is able to follow up on teaching specific tasks at home, and he learns some techniques for managing the child. He may learn to use behavior modification techniques, how to manage the environment to reduce overstimulation, to help the child shift from one activity to another without tears, and to impose a schedule and a structure on the child's daily activities.

The parent may have to become a language therapist, shortening or simplifying verbal input, and encouraging object naming, higher-level concepts, good language structure, or whatever the child needs in the area of language development.

The parent begins to feel more comfortable about his child's abilities and about his own effectiveness in dealing with him. This change in attitude on the parent's part and the changes in environment and management also produce some positive changes in the child in both learning and interpersonal relationships.

For the child who is enrolled in preschool or elementary school, reports are often sent to the school, and in some cases conferences are held. The result in most cases is an increase in understanding of the child as well as some positive steps taken to improve behavior and learning. The teacher is, more often than not, receptive to suggestions and often becomes instrumental in implementing remedial procedures.

The six children described in this chapter were referred to our clinic by alert physicians because they recognized them as having problems in acquisition of developmental skills or as being atypical in some way. None of these children are presently "cured." They have been effectively identified and diagnosed. Remedial programs have been initiated for them which improved the skills of five of the six children and helped maintain skills for the sixth. All the children benefited from the goals of the program. Their own self-concepts and ability to work independently were improved, their parents were able to manage their problems more effectively, and school-child relationships were improved.

We hope that this chapter has contributed to the understanding of the learning-disabled child and that it will be helpful in both identification and appropriate referral.

It is often a problem for the physician to know the appropriate agencies to which he can refer a child with confidence. Some of the sources he might consider include special education facilities, child development clinics, and speech and hearing clinics. The Association for Children With Learning Disabilities (ACLD) has a national directory* available which lists facilities and organizations that either diagnose and treat these children or act as referral sources.†

---

*Available from ACLD, 2200 Brownsville Road, Pittsburg, Pa. 15201.

†Another national directory of resources is the *Third Annual Directory of Facilities for the Learning Disabled,* 1970, published by Academic Therapy Publications, San Rafael, Calif. 94901.

REFERENCES

ACLD Directory, Pittsburgh, 1969, Association for Children with Learning Disabilities.

Bateman, B.: In Hellmuth, J., editor: Learning disorders, vol. 1, Seattle, 1965, Seattle Sequin School.

Beery, K. E.: Developmental test of visual-motor integration, Chicago, 1967, Follett Educational Corp.

Bender, L.: Visual-motor gestalt test and its clinical use, research monograph no. 3, New York, 1952, American Orthopsychiatric Association.

Chalfant, J. C., and Scheffeling, M. A.: Central processing dysfunction in children, Bethesda, Md., 1969, National Institutes of Health.

Cruickshank, W., editor: A teaching method for hyperactive and brain-injured children, Syracuse, 1961, Syracuse University Press.

Dunn, L.: Peabody picture vocabulary test, Nashville, 1959, American Guidance Service.

Durost, W., Bixler, H., Hildreth Co., Lund, K., and Wrightstone, J.: Metropolitan achievement tests, New York, 1959, Harcourt, Brace and World, Inc.

Fernald, G.: Remedial techniques in basic school subjects, New York, 1943, McGraw-Hill Book Co.

Fernald, G., and Keller, H.: The effect of kinesthetic factors in the development of word recognition in non-readers, J. Ed. Res. 4:355, 1921.

Frostig, M., Lefever, W., and Whittlesey, J.: Developmental test of visual perception, Palo Alto, Calif. 1966, Consulting Psychologist Press.

Gates, A. I., and McKillop, A. S.: Gates-McKillop reading diagnostic tests, New York, 1962, Teachers College Press.

Goodenough, F.: The measurement of intelligence by drawings, Yonkers-On-Hudson, N. Y., 1926, World Book Co.

Hauserman, E.: Developmental potential of preschool children, New York, 1958, Grune & Stratton, Inc.

Hellmuth, J., editor: Learning disorders, vol. 1, Seattle, 1965, Seattle Sequin School.

Johnson, D. J., and Myklebust, H.: Dyslexia in childhood. In J. Hellmuth, editor: Learning Disorders, Seattle, 1965, Special Child Publication.

Johnson, D. J., and Myklebust, H.: Learning disabilities, educational principles and practices, New York, 1967, Grune & Stratton, Inc.

Kephart, N. C.: The slow learner in the classroom, Columbus, Ohio, 1960, Charles C. Merrill Co.

Kirk, S. A.: Educating exceptional children, Boston, 1962, Houghton Mifflin Co.

McCarthy, J. J., and Kirk, S. A.: Illinois Test of Psycholinguistic Abilities, Urbana, Ill., 1961, University of Illinois Press.

Myklebust, H. R., and Boshes, B.: Minimal brain damage in children, Bethesda, Md., 1969, National Institutes of Health.

Terman, L. M., and Merrill, M. A.: Stanford-Binet Intelligence Scale; manual for the 3rd revision form L-M; with rev. IQ tables by Samuel R. Pinneau, Boston, 1960, Houghton Mifflin Co.

Third Annual Directory of Facilities for the Learning Disabled, San Rafael, Calif., 1970, Academic Therapy Publications.

Wechsler, D.: Wechsler Intelligence Scale for Children, New York, 1949, Psychological Corporation.

Wechsler, D.: Wechsler Preschool and Primary Scale of Intelligence, New York, 1967, Psychological Corp.

chapter 4

ROLE OF THE READING TEACHER
IN LEARNING DISORDERS

RICHARD W. BURNETT

At the same time that a general disaffection with public education has been growing nationally, confusion has mounted regarding how best to help children with learning problems. The incidence in the United States of public-school children who are seriously underachieving in reading is estimated to be between 10% and 20% of the white middle-class population, with an even higher incidence of failure reported among the economically deprived groups of our society. Issues are confounded by the financial plight of the schools in the face of inflation and taxpayer reluctance to vote additional taxes to support controversy-ridden schools. The militancy of teachers has increased as a result of their frustrated efforts to improve their economic position and secure a voice in decision making in education. Competition for the still immense, even though limited, funds available for the education of children has increased among groups within the educational structure itself, as well as among groups outside the schools. Amid all of this confusion the decade of the seventies has been designated by the United States Office of Education as the period for the "Right to Read" campaign. The goal is that by 1980 no schoolchild in the nation who has reached 10 years of age will be achieving in reading at a lower level than is consistent with his general mental ability. This is the backdrop against which any discussion of problems and practices in teaching reading must be cast.

The 1960's brought a multidisciplinary interest in children with school problems on a scale without precedent. Varied interest groups—medical specialists such as neurologists, psychiatrists, ophthalmologists, and pediatricians; educators, including remedial-reading teachers and those in the newly developed special education subgroups, such as teachers of the neurologically impaired, the perceptually handicapped, the minimally brain-damaged, and the academically maladjusted, and the ubiquitous learning disability specialists; psychologists; guidance counselors; optometrists; physical therapists; and others—all have attempted to respond to the growing clamor from organizations of distraught parents who are pressing for immediate assistance for children having difficulties in school. With this divergence of interest, it is not at all strange that some of the explanations for learning problems and the related suggestions for correction appear largely incompatible with one another.

Among the earlier entrants into the field of diagnosing and treating learning disorders were the reading specialists, who have maintained since the early 1930's a record of research, testing and treatment procedure, and a university curriculum for training modest numbers of remedial reading teachers in an internship setting at the graduate school level. In the next pages an attempt will be made to develop a "reading point of view" in looking at the current complex and confusing area of learning disorders.

WHAT IS READING AND WHY IS IT TAUGHT IN SCHOOL?

Have you ever tried to define *thinking* in a manner that would be helpful to those interested in effectively teaching others to do it? Like thinking, *reading* is one of those developmental processes which are difficult to define because of their changing characteristics within maturing individuals. Some definitions of reading are shallow and superficial because those who pose them are so obviously seeing only one facet of the total process. A complete definition may seem cumbersome and obtuse, but the effort to develop one is a necessary element in all dialogue about reading. It may be helpful to begin by considering reading as one application of a broader set of language skills that include oral and aural language. Just as listening is receptive language, or the decoding side of the expressive, or encoding, ability we call speech, reading is the decoding side of writing. As a communication process, reading encompasses sensory, perceptual, and cognitive aspects, all operating simultaneously in an individual's deliberate effort to secure another person's ideas recorded in printed symbol form.

In our culture, reading is extremely important, assuming a role almost as essential to a modern individual as the ability to understand oral language or communicate through speech. To be able to read is even more important than to be able to communicate effectively through writing. Just as with listening proficiency or speaking effectiveness, there are tremendous individual differences in the facility with which individuals can read. A complicating factor in reading, beyond those subskills called for in listening to ideas and understanding and retaining them, is the mediating step required in turning visually received printed symbols into oral language symbols to which meaning is attached. In the classroom the subskills in this mediating step are called word recognition skills. The relative ease with which children acquire the word recognition skills is the factor that brings about the greatest differentiation in achievement at the beginning stages of academic learning. Some few individuals acquire these word recognition skills and raise them to an automatic level of operation without any systematic efforts having been made to teach them. On the other hand, some do not pick up this ability to turn visual symbols into oral language, and these learners founder at or near the very beginning stages of learning to read. It is precisely for this reason—that reading is not readily acquired through inductive learning or picked up incidentally as other language functions are—that reading is formally taught in school.

In today's society a child's speech and listening facility are commonly assumed to be influenced as much through other environmental conditions as they are through school learning experiences. Not so with reading. Since the school accepts the responsibility to introduce reading, the school is charged with having failed when individuals do not acquire facility in reading that is consistent with the performance standard for the group. As a consequence the number one priority in the primary grades of the school is to get the pupils off to a successful start in reading.

HOW IS READING TAUGHT?

In our traditional school programs, children are expected to learn to read in the following manner. In kindergarten and early first grade, efforts are taken to ensure that children known the meanings of common words and are able to distinguish the sound elements that make up spoken words. Then they are exposed to printed words and taught that these stand for concepts they know. As a child becomes aware of differences in the appearance of printed words, he is taught that specific visual symbols stand for specific sounds, and he is expected to generalize from words with which he has had repeated experience to the analysis of words he has not previously met. In a good reading program, a considerable amount of review, reteaching, and overlearning of the basic principles is provided throughout the primary grades, first grade through third grade. After third grade the emphasis on the mechanical aspects of reading—sounding principles leading to the pronunciation of words—gives way to an increasing emphasis on understanding and interpreting what is being read. After third grade the child who has not mastered the mechanical skills is less and less likely, as he progresses through the grades, to be taught by teachers who are trained to teach these skills or who are interested in teaching the basic mechanical skills of reading.

Dating back to the McGuffey *Eclectic Readers* of the middle nineteenth century, the classic way to maintain reading instruction for a pupil throughout the grades has been to place printed material in his hands that (1) was presumed to be interesting to him, (2) was presented in a vocabulary that did not overtax his mechanical reading skills, so that he could recognize most words, and (3) contained concepts within his range of understanding. While guiding the pupil's reading of these materials to accomplish some purpose, such as securing information or simply enjoying a good story, the teacher has been expected to improve the learner's word recognition skills, expand his vocabulary, and develop his ability to comprehend what he reads. Heavily emphasized in earlier times, but with generally less emphasis today, was much reading aloud from the story anthologies, and a major objective was to develop oral language facility as part of the reading program. Directions to the teacher were aimed at bringing about expressive oral readers who practiced acceptable patterns of pronunciation, expression, and voice projection. Today's emphasis is more on the development of independent silent reading ability, and even where oral reading is done, the objective is often improvement in silent reading while using oral activity to monitor the learner's progress in acquiring the skills essential for reading fluency.

For about the last twenty-five years, word recognition has been defined as that aspect of reading which encompasses the learner's use of (1) sight words, that is, words responded to instantly without resorting to deliberate analysis; (2) context clues; (3) word analysis, including both phonic and structural, with phonic analysis being a sounding approach, whereas structural analysis is a visual approach to dividing words into elements; and (4) the dictionary, which requires being able to locate a given word, pronounce it, and come up with the appropriate definition. The word recognition skills have been called the "mechanical skills" of reading in contrast to the comprehension skills, or "higher reading skills," which are concerned with the understanding of ideas once the printed words are translated into oral language.

The crux of nearly all the controversies over how to teach reading is found in the haggling over how best to teach children the word recognition skills. Some approaches stress teaching children to see words as collections of individual letters, each of which must be sounded out. Other approaches stress teaching children to resort to a variety of ways of recognizing words, depending on the context in which the word is found, the pattern of its spelling, or the structural elements in its makeup. In some programs, it is assumed that all children will learn on first exposure, and the skills are taught at a rapid pace and early in the beginning stages of school. In other programs, the pace is measured and slow, much repetition is built in, and the same skills may be reintroduced in a number of ways. Modes of presentation vary, with some approaches counting heavily on ear training, others on visual learning, and some on a deliberate balance of visual and auditory training. Still others require motor involvement of the learner through an earlier and greater emphasis on writing than is usual with other approaches.

It is a truism to say that at least a simple majority of children in any typical group are likely to learn to read through the enthusiastic teaching of any method ever conceived. It is also true, unfortunately, that a certain percentage of the children will fail to learn at a pace consistent with the majority no matter what approach, materials, or techniques are used. As the beginning approaches vary, the children who fail to respond to instruction will vary, at least to some degree. As these pupils fall behind significantly, and the instruction in the classroom is not able to keep them progressing properly, corrective or remedial reading help may be provided. It should be noted, however, that there has never been a time in American schools when remedial reading help was available for more than a small minority of those who appeared to need it. Effective remedial efforts approach greater specificity than most classroom teaching in finding the points of breakdown in a learner's overall reading functioning and in developing the weak subskill areas. The remedial teacher is expected to be attuned to the varieties of ways in which given skills might be developed and is better able to match the proper approach and materials of instruction to the learner than is possible in the group instruction of the regular classroom.

HOW IS REMEDIAL READING RELATED TO CLASSROOM INSTRUCTION?

In the jargon of the special reading teacher, the overall effort of the school to develop reading facility in all students is called the *developmental* reading program. The developmental program is all-encompassing in that it includes all pupils and all teachers at all grade levels. Since the instruction in the classroom is directed to groups in which there is a wide range of differences among individual learners, it is expected that some may need special instruction to keep up with the group standard. The program of instruction offered to selected groups in an effort to help them "catch up" so that they can progress with the larger group is called the *corrective* reading program. Despite the best efforts within the school to teach some children to read in group settings, there are still some who fail to progress. A third kind of instructional program is the *remedial* reading program, which is meant to be reserved for learners unable to profit from group instructional efforts and is offered on a one-to-one, teacher-to-learner basis, or as nearly so as possible.

Reflection on the three kinds of school reading programs makes it clear that the extent and nature of remedial reading help is dependent on the relative effectiveness of the corrective efforts. In turn, the nature and extent of the corrective program rests on the relative quality of the developmental reading program. As better informed teachers learn how to alleviate problems before they become severe and to maintain individual progress in the group instructional setting, the extent of special corrective and remedial efforts should diminish. In some school settings, classroom teachers are asked to participate in a year of remedial reading work under supervision as a means of equipping them to teach problem learners more effectively after returning to the classroom.

The reading specialist is the first to recognize that extensive remedial reading programs are not the hallmark of a good school reading program. Rather, a school reading program of excellence is one in which close coordination exists between classroom developmental teaching, corrective reading groups, and the remedial reading efforts. This coordinated effort is felt to offer the most effective program for the individual with learning problems, as well as to lead to the best possible instruction for groups of normal learners. Classroom teachers should know the instructional strategy and materials used with those pupils in their classes who are receiving special instruction outside the classroom. Furthermore, corrective and remedial teachers should know the demands placed on their pupils when they are in the regular classroom and thus be in a position to play a supportive role. There should be a mutual reinforcement of efforts to teach the child with learning problems on the part of all who are working with him. Where there is no communication or integration of the collective efforts to teach, optimal learning experiences for the pupil cannot be maintained.

Steps have been taken by the reading teachers to bring about the implementation of this concept of a coordinated program for children with reading disabilities. For more than ten years the International Reading Association has fought to maintain reading specialization as a graduate-degree specialty, in contrast, for example, to speech correctionists or special education teachers, who are commonly trained in undergraduate programs and certificated at the bachelor's-degree level. The special reading teacher is expected to have been a successful classroom teacher who has acquired additional training and experience beyond that of the usual classroom teacher. His role includes serving as a consultant and resource person for other teachers, helping them to improve their classroom group instruction, while at the same time he is working with the more seriously underachieving children. A reading specialist is expected to be familiar with the varieties of instructional programs and materials that compete with each other for adoption in the classroom. He is expected to know the underlying rationale for these programs and the correlated materials, and how to make best use of them in meeting individual differences in the large-group setting. By understanding the developmental-reading offering, he is better able to relate corrective and remedial efforts to it in a way that strengthens the overall instructional program.

Reading specialists have resisted the trend to stamp underachievers in reading with labels that imply that these pupils are not "normal" or that they are exceptional children who must be segregated wholly, or even for a substantial portion of their schooling, from the mainstream of education. The divisiveness among specialists in the "learning disabilities" movement that gained momentum in the 1960's is one reason for the reluctance of remedial reading teachers to lend their unqualified support to it. The development of a professional jargon based on several competitive theoretical formulations that are both loosely contrived and untested by time or controlled research studies could be a step backward in serving the needs of large numbers of underachieving children in American schools. To support special educational programs that are manned by persons untrained and inexperienced as classroom elementary teachers, and that are administered and financed, in many instances, outside the regular school district, may be to impede or preclude altogether the evolution of an integrated instructional offering, combining developmental, corrective, and remedial efforts in the attempt to meet the needs of the child with a specific learning deficit.

HOW DOES THE READING TEACHER APPROACH LEARNING DISABILITIES?

In reading clinics and remedial reading programs a child is seldom seen for whom some effort has not been made to teach him to read. The basis for his referral, of course, is that he has not responded to instruction as well as expected, in the judgment of the one making the referral. Where the referral is appropriate and the child is underachieving, the goal of a remedial program is to equip him with some functional reading proficiency as soon as possible. If he has some proficiency already, the goal is to show him how to make better use of it and to improve it to the level where his reading better serves him in meeting the demands placed on him in and out of school. Other considerations are of secondary concern. The reading teacher's attitude toward testing and treatment must be assessed in the context of his commitment to success in reading as a major behavioral objective.

In one observer's analysis reading remediation might be categorized as visual-motor perception training because of the reading teacher's effort to train the child to use visual cues in letter and word discrimination and to develop in the child a left-to-right orientation in visual scanning. On the other hand, another observer, believing that an emotional disturbance is the basis for learning problems, might call the same remediation effort psychotherapeutic because of the reading teacher's acceptance of the child's level of performance, his effort to assure initial success, his magnification of every gain, his effort to appeal to the child's intrinsic interests by selecting certain instructional activities and materials, and his care in not allowing the pupil to feel that he is being compared unfavorably to others. Unlike the vague and diffuse objectives of some visual-motor perception strategies and of some behavioral modification efforts offered under the banner of "learning disabilities" programs, the objective in reading remediation is clearly defined, and the payoff is direct and evident in the child's improved reading performance.

In a remedial reading setting the following questions are the basis of the diagnosis:

1. What is the pupil's current reading level?
2. At what level should he be reading?
3. Is he a disabled reader?
4. Are there any outside factors contributing to his problem?
5. What are his skill strengths and weaknesses?
6. What recommendations are in order to improve his deficit, and who should implement them?

Reading testing

The first question regarding the pupil's reading level is not as clear-cut as might be assumed, since reading is measurable in so many ways. A standardized reading test may be administered in which the reader answers multiple-choice questions. His number of correct responses is compared to the results from a large sample population and reported in a grade-level score. Although such tests are very adequate devices for measuring achievement gains in large groups, in individual cases the results may be distorted. A pupil may be adept at matching words without being able to read at all. As a consequence he may earn a score significantly higher than the level at which he can actually function. In other words, a child scoring a 3.2 grade equivalent on many reading tests might not be able to read fluently at third-grade or even first-grade level. To establish how well a reader can function, the examiner may ask him to read aloud from material of differing grade levels. The same type of material may be given to him to read silently also. With the use of both silently and orally read materials, questions are asked to check for comprehension and recall. It is well to remember that the degree of comprehension is often related to the types of questions asked. The direct, detail type of question produces better results than a general question, such as "Can you tell me what you read?" In a complete reading analysis, reading is assessed by several methods before a judgment is made about an individual's reading proficiency.

A final, related note about measuring reading achievement is that in any research in which gains in reading are reported as a result of a particular treatment, a distinction must be made between a statistically significant increase in the number of correct responses on a standardized test, and improvement in reading as demonstrated by the ability to read more difficult material with better fluency and comprehension. In the first instance, individuals can be taught to respond to items similar to those on the test and thus be made to appear to have achieved dramatic growth in reading in a short time. Some commercial remedial reading programs that guarantee specified results within a time limit simply provide practice with the types of questions appearing on the testing instruments used before and after the programs are conducted. This kind of cynicism is also evident in many adult basic education programs and literacy projects in which the method of raising individuals to a "high school graduate's level of functioning" in six to ten weeks is often based on the repeated testing of enrollees until they finally score at the required level.

The reason for raising the question as to the level at which the pupil *should* be reading is that age or grade placement alone is not a valid basis for stating the level at which a learner should be achieving. Usually a mental age based on an individually administered intelligence test is the basis for stating what the reading performance ought to be. This capacity index must be related, of course, to the opportunity a pupil has had to learn. A child of normal intelligence who is in the fourth grade at the age of 9 years would be expected to read better than a similar child of the same age and IQ who is only in grade 3. However, a 9-year-old child who is in the fourth grade and has an IQ of 80 would not be expected to be doing any better in reading than a younger child who is in the third grade and has an IQ of 120.

Another informal device sometimes used to determine whether capacity to learn is above actual functioning in reading is the comparing of the most difficult reading passage the pupil can understand when he reads it with the most difficult passage he can understand when it is read to him. If a fourth-grade pupil cannot read a second-grade passage but can understand material of fifth-grade difficulty when it is read aloud to him, he is clearly a disabled reader. In contrast, a fourth grader who can neither read a second-grade passage nor understand it when it is read aloud to him has a problem other than reading.

Visual testing

If it is determined that a significant discrepancy exists between reading achievement and predicted reading level, the next effort is to find out if any outside factors are contributing to the deficiency. Visual acuity is checked, usually through the use of an instrument such as a Bausch & Lomb Ortho-Rater or a Keystone Telebinocular. If the child's vision is inadequate in either eye or both eyes at near or far point, his parents will be asked to take the child to a vision specialist for an examination and possible correction. Normally, direct referrals are not made, and parents are expected to select their own ophthalmologist or optometrist. The judgment of the specialist is not questioned in regard to the prescription of corrective lenses. If lenses have been prescribed, the pupil is expected to wear them for all testing and instruction. The uncertainty as to how a child will be received by a vision specialist if he shows only a possible deficiency in phoria or depth perception usually prevents referral for these conditions unless acuity is also impaired.

If the child does appear to have a vision problem, special attention is paid during testing and in the early periods of remedial teaching to the extent to which the condition seems to be contributing to the reading difficulty. Areas of concern include the following: Does he resist reading for more than a few minutes at a time? Does he squint or hold his eyes unusually near to or far from the printed page? Does his accuracy in pronouncing words appear to be related to changes in type size? The obvious modifications in instructional procedures recommended might include keeping instructional periods short and offering them more frequently, varying work done at near point with chalkboard work, and using books with larger type.

Other therapy

Hearing is usually screened by means of a pure-tone air-conduction audiometer, and referral to a medical specialist is recommended to the parents when significantly acuity deficits are uncovered. Modifications in teaching are made when a hearing deficit is believed to be interfering with the child's auditory discrimination.

Other areas of possible importance often investigated to some degree include unusual behavior patterns, which indicate either physical or psychological problems. Acting-out behavior in school or at home, sleeping and eating habits, enuresis, school attendance pattern, home conditions, health records, and developmental history are examined in a clinical setting as well as in many public school remedial reading programs. Such factors, although not generally the single cause of a reading deficit, are identified as "inhibiting" factors. Occasionally, insight into how best to instruct a particular child results from a study of the complex of factors impinging on his school performance.

Of primary importance to the reading-oriented therapist is the careful analysis of a pupil's skill strengths and weaknesses. A first effort is the identification of the level of performance in reading in order to establish the type of reading the pupil can be expected to do while working to improve himself. The level of difficulty of the material must be such that the pupil is able to read with fair fluency and comprehension when working under the guidance of a teacher. Often in testing the pupil with a severe disability, there is no such level. Then the effort is to pinpoint as accurately as possible what the problem reader can do. Areas to be explored include the following: Does he recognize any words at sight? How many? Does he understand the use of context clues to assist him in reading? Does he make use of the general length or shape of words at all in trying to read them? Does he use beginning letters? Ending letters? Middle letters? If not, does he know the letters of the alphabet? The sounds for which they stand? Can he point to the letter when it is named? When its sound is given? Can he match letters or words that are the same?

When the child exhibits negligible knowledge of these reading subskills, prognostic lessons may be taught to establish whether he can be taught to name letters, discriminate sounds in words, associate sounds with letters, and respond to a few sight words after several exposures.

At somewhat higher levels of performance the pupil may exhibit a sizable sight vocabulary and good use of context clues but may be weak in word analysis skills when the material has a high proportion of words with which he has not had previous experience. Some students, especially those of normal to above-average mental ability, pick up sight words so readily and use context clues so well that their inability to pronounce previously unlearned words may go unnoticed in the group instruction until they are fairly well along in the school grades. When the reading load increases dramatically in the middle grades, this type of deficit may cause them to become underachievers, apparently without warning, much to the dismay of the children, their parents, and their teachers. Normally, if the cause of the children's sudden floundering is identified, specific instruction of fairly short duration aimed at their deficit can keep them from becoming severely handicapped.

Some experienced reading teachers make a distinction between "hard core" reading problems and "garden variety" problems. The garden variety are the ones that respond quickly to short-term remedial assistance, and the students are able to return to classroom instruction without special supportive help. The "hard core" problems do not respond to remedial efforts of short duration. Extended efforts are needed to teach the coding features of written or printed language. The children with these problems are the ones who are subjected to the myriad labels offered by various groups of specialists. From a reading teacher's point of view, what is needed for these children is a continuing effort to provide reading experiences at their level of performance, whatever it is and regardless of their grade placement. At this reading level, the specific skills not yet mastered must be taught, often in a manner or variety of manners differing from the approach normally used in group instruction in the classroom. While these pupils receive reading help at a lower level than their grade placement, they must continue to remain in classes with their peers, where special efforts are made to assist them to keep up in background knowledge, new concepts, and information through listening or through any avenue other than reading, including observing demonstrations, viewing films, or having direct experience through field trips.

Recommendations coming out of a reading diagnosis are usually directed to the classroom teacher and the remedial teacher, with the children having the most severe deficits receiving a greater share of remedial efforts, and those with less severe deficiency receiving less remedial attention. Remedial reading teachers, typically, are oriented to "make do" with whatever space or resources are made available to them. Since schools are overcrowded and underfinanced, and space is at a premium in most school buildings throughout the United States, remedial reading is often offered in boiler rooms, hallways, nurses' offices, supply rooms, and other makeshift quarters. Materials and instructional supplies are usually limited. Maintaining class schedules around lunch and physical education training is often given higher priority by both classroom teachers and building administrators than the scheduling of remedial or corrective instruction. It would be foolish to pretend that optimal remedial instruction is available in most public schools of our nation. It simply is not. If remedial reading has failed, as some contend who are pressing for new models for educational "intervention" for children with school learning disabilities, its failure lies in its efforts to work as efficiently as possible within the system rather than setting up peripheral programs.

WHAT IS THE READING TEACHER'S ATTITUDE TOWARD DYSLEXIA?

The term "dyslexia" is abhorrent to most reading teachers, just as it is to many medical practitioners, because it implies the existence of a condition which, at the present time and on a rational basis, it is perfectly legitimate to deny exists at all. The term "dyslexia" in circles where it is acceptable and correctly used can be applied only to a *normal* child or, infrequently, adult who is unable to learn to read with the facility expected despite optimal efforts to teach him. By "normal" is meant intelligence in the average or above-average range, intact senses, the motivation to learn, and emotional adjustment within reasonable limits. Medically, dyslexia would be an *idiopathic* condition, since its cause is unknown. Furthermore, it would be *chronic,* since there is no known cure, and spontaneous remission or recovery is unknown. Dyslexia is a debilitating condition only when certain conditions external to the patient are present. This last point is important, since in some cultures, even in subcultures within our own country, dyslexia has no meaning or at least a different meaning from that which it has in another strata of our society. Until the recent past, the condition called dyslexia has been limited almost exclusively to children from white, middle-class homes where standard English was spoken.

It is further ironic that not only can the condition termed dyslexia not be diagnosed medically, but it cannot be treated medically. A physician, be he neurologist, psychiatrist, ophthalmologist, or pediatrician, can apply the label with any degree of honesty only after he is assured that a patient is failing to learn to read despite the school's best efforts to teach him. Reading teachers generally welcome all the help they can get in working with children who are unable to acquire reading facility with ease, but they regret the obfuscation that diffuses such help with the application of a label such as dyslexia.

WHAT NEEDS TO BE DONE?

In the 1970's attention in American schools will be concentrated on those pupils of normal mental ability who display specific learning disorders that interfere with their fully profiting from the available educational opportunities. Few question the existence of unconscionably large numbers of such pupils, and fewer still argue against the mounting of programs designed to decrease the incidence of learning disorders and provide optimal education for those who are disabled learners. Although serious and legitimate differences of opinion do exist over issues such as the causes of learning disorders and rational classification schemes, the greatest concern is over assuring that the most effective strategies for educational therapy are initiated immediately. As with any "crash program" efforts, development and refinement of the problem-solving strategy take place in a climate where the major share of resources and energy is directed to resolving the problem. It is still early enough in the learning disabilities movement to caution against the ultimate direction that early precipitous action might take and to suggest that there are different and perhaps more direct routes to accomplishing the same ends.

Some observers, including this one, see the situation in the following light: As our technological society makes it increasingly less possible to provide suitable employment and satisfactory life adjustment opportunities for the adult having a low level of literacy, parents and professionals concerned with the education of children have become increasingly anxious over the numbers of those who are not responding to instruction. Pressure brought to bear on government at both federal and state levels has resulted in an increase in the amount of funds available to use in establishing programs to aid those who are perceived as not learning properly. Varied "intervention" strategies have been formulated, based on the idea that if these pupils are identified, diagnosed, and subsequently treated in some special way for an undetermined period of time, they can be returned to the "mainstream" of education and maintain normal progress. These programs vary widely in underlying rationale, the nature of their diagnostic and treatment procedures, and the extent to which they are compatible or even seek to be compatible with other educational programs and classroom procedures. Complicating the implementation of fruitful instructional programs for children with specific learning disorders is the looseness of this particular classification. Medical, psychological, and special educational efforts directed toward the analysis and treatment of children unequivocally diagnosed as brain-damaged, autistic, schizophrenic, or otherwise emotionally disturbed have too often been carried beyond reasonable delimitations and have influenced the diagnostic labeling and therapeutic strategies suggested for much less severely handicapped children.

Wherever euphemisms are coined by persons interested in the child with specific learning problems, the basis of the impairment, for the large majority of these children, is that they cannot read and do not respond to the instruction offered in the classroom group setting. Just as some children appear not to be able to learn to play a violin, or just as some adults, after years of practice and expensive lessons, cannot play a round of par golf, it is plausible to suggest that some otherwise perfectly normal children cannot acquire reading skills with the ease and at the pace that the majority of children can. Unfortunately for these "normal" children, they live at a time when reading weakness or failure cannot be tolerated, and in addition, they are enrolled in schools that are basically assembly-line operations. The harried adults trying to run the factories—teachers and school administrators —welcome all too frequently the evasion of responsibility that ensues when it is suggested that children who do not learn are failing because of deficits within the child rather than within the educational system. Often these children are seen as an embarrassment by their families as well as the school personnel, and the effects of the consequent punitive measures are incalculable in terms of the damage wrought upon the child. Examples include staying in from recess for "special" help, "flunking" first grade or any other grade, no television viewing permitted at home, the endless round of diagnostic referrals, the phonics records and kits advertised in magazine and newspapers and foisted off on the child by a nearly hysterical parent, and the year-after-year assignment of failing and almost failing grades in all aspects of the curriculum related to reading. It is no wonder that when these children are examined by different specialists, they are perceived to have such a confusing array of symptoms—hyperactivity, tics, anxiety, depression, perceptual-motor deficits, linguistic irregularities, enuresis, "soft" neurological signs, etc.

The following observations, from a reading teacher's point of view, should be taken into account in furthering efforts to decrease the incidence of learning disorders as well as to bring aid to children who presently have these disorders:

1. Parents, educators, and other interested professionals must recognize that the best possible programs of instruction in the schools will result in some otherwise normal and healthy children not learning to read at a pace consistent with that at which their peers learn.

2. Reading problems in children must be looked at from a societal, or cultural, perspective. In ordinary circumstances, a child's ability or inability to read should not be seen as any more of a medical concern than an individual's ability to play a violin or play par golf except that our society puts such a high premium on reading proficiency early in a child's development.

3. Practices involving the application of labels such as congenital dyslexia or developmental dyslexia, minimal brain dysfunction, or perceptual-motor im-

pairment to physiologically normal children having difficulties in acquiring reading skills are to be discouraged, since these practices impart an aura of legitimacy to a type of differential diagnosis that at the present time is impossible to make and that is sometimes used to support therapeutic strategies that have little or no educational merit.

4. Efforts within the schools to better meet the problem must be supported. A necessary step is the elimination of the concept that the only way to conduct schools is to close one adult in a room with twenty to thirty children. At the very least, placing a teacher aide in every elementary classroom should be considered in order to make it possible for teachers to implement those individualized instructional practices with which many of them are familiar but which they are unable to use because of the pressures of constantly working alone with a group.

5. Reading instruction at each pupil's level of development must be maintained throughout his school attendance. At the same time, for the reader achieving below grade level, opportunities to keep up in vocabulary development, background information, and new concepts must be provided through learning experiences based on avenues other than reading.

chapter 5

EDUCATION FOR CHILDREN WITH LEARNING DISABILITIES

ELEANORE T. KENNEY

BACKGROUND AND DEFINITION
Historical background—interdisciplinary interest

Within the past decade, since the early 1960's, special educators have turned increasing attention to the child of normal intellect who is unable to learn in school. Among these children are a number frequently diagnosed as dyslexic, that is, as having major problems related to the reception of written symbols, with a primary difficulty in learning to read. The understanding of diagnostic and remedial needs of the dyslexic child is immeasurably enriched and helped by a knowledge of educational approaches used with children with other kinds of learning disabilities.

Still other children, within the range of normal intellect, have different kinds of specific learning disabilities that severely handicap achievement in school. The learning disability movement has stimulated innovative and varied educational approaches to diagnosing problems and planning curricula to help such children compensate for these many kinds of disorders, including the particular problems related to dyslexia. The focus of this chapter will be on past and current developments in diagnosis and education of children with varied kinds of learning disorders.

The educational literature about children with specific learning disabilities has mushroomed in recent years. In this literature there is no clear professional unanimity on the meaning of the term "learning disability." The definitions have factors common to all but differ with respect to emphasis on biological and/or psychological factors. Differences seem to be related to the professional discipline involved and the vocabulary relevant to that particular profession.

A definition that assists understanding and helps to overcome differences in terminology between the medical profession and educators is that used in the Children With Specific Learning Disabilities Act of 1969. This definition was originally recommended by the National Advisory Committee on the Handicapped:

> The term 'children with specific learning disabilities' means those children who have a disorder in one or more of the basic psychological processes involved in under-

standing or in using language, spoken or written, which disorder may manifest itself in imperfect ability to listen, think, speak, read, write, spell, or do mathematical calculations. Such disorders include conditions such as perceptual handicaps, brain injury, minimal brain dysfunction, dyslexia, and developmental aphasia. Such term does not include children who have learning problems which are primarily the result of visual, hearing, or motor handicaps, of mental retardation, of emotional disturbance, or of environmental disadvantage.

It is not surprising in the history of special education that the identification of special needs of children began with the most grossly apparent handicaps, that is, crippling, blindness, and deafness. Then came the focus on the retarded child, who in many instances appears physically normal but has a marked discrepancy in cognitive ability compared to that of the child in the average range of intelligence. It is only within recent years that the child of normal intelligence who also has no apparent physical defect, but who has been unable to learn, has become the focus of attention. Two main divisions of special education have developed for such children: (1) programs to help children of normal intelligence who are emotionally disturbed, labeled ED programs, (2) programs for children of normal intelligence who have learning disabilities, labeled LD programs.

Prior to 1960 professional interest in helping emotionally disturbed youngsters was clinical rather than educational in beliefs and goals. There was minimal interest in educational and teaching techniques per se. Instead, the focus was on developing a therapeutic milieu, based on a therapeutic philosophy derived from the experiences of psychiatrists and clinical psychologists involved in child guidance clinics or in residential treatment settings. In contrast, initial interests, at different points in time, in planning educationally for learning-disabled children came from many disciplines: neurology, psychology, optometry, remedial reading, and speech and hearing. In view of this mixed heritage it is quite understandable that the learning-disabled child has had many labels attached to him, with varied emphasis, such as etiological terminology (brain damage, minimal cerebral dysfunction), terminology pinpointing the deficit in a particular sensory process (perceptual-motor), labels of certain symbol dysfunctions (dyslexia), and terminology determining the functional levels of such specific abilities as listening, thinking, remembering, talking, reading, writing, spelling, and doing arithmetic.

Inasmuch as the concern of this chapter is primarily educational, only functional and process terms will be used, with no elaboration of neurological etiology. From an educational point of view, it is improper for a term such as "brain damage" or "minimal cerebral dysfunction" to be entered on a child's school record. This is not to say that the study of etiology is unimportant. To the contrary, it is of great consequence to the learning disability movement. As more refined diagnostic methods develop, the day may arrive when correlated patterns of central process dysfunctions are more clearly understood from a neurological point of view. When these patterns are thus clarified, it may conceivably then be possible to correlate them with observable behavior patterns, which are the primary concern of the educator.

The reader interested in exploring neurological literature will find an extensive discussion and annotated bibliography on etiology in Birch. Birch sees the term "brain damage" not as representing a neurological entity but rather as describing a behavior pattern. However, many children with a learning disability (hereafter termed LD) do not give evidence of damage as determined by standard neurological tests. Instead, tests of perception and psychological tests are needed for purposes of educational diagnosis.

Number and types of LD children

As the learning disability concept developed, attempts have been made to estimate the prevalence of children who would fit into such a category. In view of the broad range of children that might be included in the definition of the 1969 learning disabilities act, it is not surprising that estimates have ranged from 5% to 20% of the school-age population. Many more boys than girls have difficulties, and the male-female ratio is five to one. In making these estimates we suspect many children have been diagnosed as having specific learning disabilities who have instead been taught in the wrong manner. Such children should be said to have educational disabilities rather than learning disabilities arising from constitutional deficits.

Adelman (1971) hypothesizes that among the LD population there are children with three major kinds of learning problems, which he designates as types I, II, and III disorders. Children with type III are the hard-core "specific learning disability" children who have major learning process disorders. Type II are those youngsters who have minor learning process disorders but, given appropriate learning environments, can readily compensate for such disorders. Type I are those children whose learning problem is entirely due to poor learning environments.

Consequently, Adelman holds that children with types I and II disorders are educationally handicapped, having problems largely caused by poor teaching and curriculum planning, rather than due to any disorder inherent in the child. We would agree that the term "specific learning disability" should be applied only to the type III disorder, and youngsters with the lesser types of disabilities would best be considered educationally handicapped.

It is significant that the Congress of the United States officially recognized the handicaps of these children in the writing of the Children With Specific Learning Disabilities Act of 1969. This legislation has resulted in the implementation of varied kinds of public school programs throughout the United States, and it is also prompting the development of teacher training programs that will graduate special education teachers who can carry out personalized diagnostic teaching in both special and regular school settings.

As the many disciplines involved with these various populations of children become more knowledgeable, it will be possible to make finer and finer distinctions among and within these subgroups. The educational importance of making these distinctions cannot be overemphasized. The goal is to maximize the use of manpower and money in the effort to ensure that LD children realize their maximum intellectual potential. Educators have much to learn in this regard, and schools are a long way from being able to diagnose children with disorders on the basis of the categories of types I, II, and III. However, educational theory and practices have been increasingly clarified since the early 1960's, when the learning disability concept became crystallized by Kirk. The diagnostic and curriculum ideas generated by the learning disability concept are challenging and show promise of creating a healthy ferment that could lead to a "new look" in both regular and special education.

PSYCHO-EDUCATIONAL DIAGNOSIS OF LEARNING DISABILITIES

At this point in time the diagnosis of learning disabilities is highly dependent on a clinically sensitive piecing together of many facets of observed and measured behavior. The immediate goal of such a diagnosis is to determine the child's strengths and weaknesses in varied combinations of visual-motor and auditory-verbal processes as well as to analyze his academic skill strengths and weaknesses. The ultimate goal is for the diagnosis to yield useful and specific knowledge that can be directly related to helping teachers who are involved with the child plan and implement a remedial program that will enable him to compensate for his disabilities.

To realize this ultimate goal, many disciplines will be involved, with a necessary backdrop of knowledge gained from medical examinations, including physical, neurological, and ophthalmological examinations. The educator's focus is on educational behavioral analysis. Ideally, medical, psychological, speech and hearing, and educational experts are in a team setting, making it possible to integrate all the diagnostic parts for the school personnel who are directly involved on a day-to-day basis with the child.

In some clinic settings throughout the country this kind of team approach is possible and is carried out. More often than not, however, this is not the case. Special services vary from school district to school district, and full medical or clinical coverage is not available in many communities. The focus here will be directed toward the three component parts of the educational behavioral analysis: psychological evaluation, language evaluation, and academic evaluation. These three areas encompass all the aspects that should be considered as a psycho-educational diagnosis is made. Just which professional disciplines, in or out of the school system, may carry out the various parts of the total evaluation will depend on the local community situation.

Psychological evaluation

Psychological diagnostic skills for identifying LD children are not definitive at this point of knowledge. The clinical psychologist evaluates, by means of behavioral observation and individually administered tests, the intellectual potential and level of emotional development of the child. In determining whether a child has a specific learning disability, the psychologist begins by finding out the problems he does *not* have. Through the process of elimination he rules out mental retardation and primary emotional disturbance as causes for learning difficulties in school.

In making these differential diagnoses, the clinician analyzes in depth the scatter of observed and measured behavior patterns of the child. The examiner appraises sensory strengths and weaknesses by determining the kinds of tasks a child can and cannot do. Such an analysis of the child's responses to a battery of standardized tests allows the clinician to compare what a particular child can and cannot do with respect to what a child of his age should be able to do.

In the instance of the LD child, there will frequently prove to be many skills that measure in the average to superior range, joined with varied below-average to retarded skills. The clinician looks for a pattern of weaknesses and strengths in the learning process. Does the child receive information better through auditory or through visual channels? Does he abstract and/or associate thoughts better on a visual or an auditory basis? Does he express himself better verbally, motorically through gesture, or in writing? In conceptualizing this pattern of how a child's mind works, it is helpful for the clinician to use the learning process model set forth in Fig. 5-1. This input-association-output model delineates the sense modalities through which a child learns about the world around him (input); the way in which he stores information (memory) so that he can build up language and thought processes (association); and the manner in which he is able to express these thoughts (output) to the adults and children in his world.

By the time a child reaches school age he is dependent largely on visual and auditory channels to receive and interpret information about the world around him. Earlier infant and preschool learning depends on the more primitive sensory mechanisms of smell, taste, touch, and kinesthetic input experiences. The psychologist has tests that help him sort out the input sensory strengths and weaknesses of a child. Thus he determines whether there are receptive difficulties. Additional tests determine whether memory difficulties are present. Examples of the kinds of test items used to assess immediate and delayed memory skills are given in Fig. 5-1.

A further analysis of the child's learning processes in the associative areas is made possible through the quantitative and qualitative assessment of all subtest measures that relate to varied dimensions of thinking and abstracting processes, as outlined in the sample items listed in Fig. 5-1. Still other tests enable the psychologist to determine the child's best channels of expression, that is, motor, oral, or written.

The analysis of test results within the framework of the input-association-output model enables a clinician to assess roughly wherein the learning process has been short-circuited and to generate a remediation plan for the teacher. Both diagnosti-

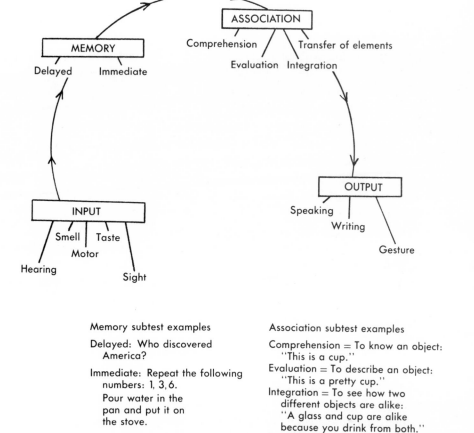

Memory subtest examples

Delayed: Who discovered America?

Immediate: Repeat the following numbers: 1, 3, 6.
Pour water in the pan and put it on the stove.

Association subtest examples

Comprehension = To know an object: "This is a cup."

Evaluation = To describe an object: "This is a pretty cup."

Integration = To see how two different objects are alike: "A glass and cup are alike because you drink from both."

Transfer of elements = To understand a concept by recognizing common elements and parts in objects: "Cupness" and "boxness" are equal to concept of "container."

FIG. 5-1. Model of the learning process.

cian and teacher come to see the many dimensions that compose a given child's intellectual potential for learning. In this manner clusters of weaknesses in the learning process are isolated. It is hypothesized that these weaknesses are correlated with, and perhaps contribute to, poor academic achievement. A teaching plan is then devised to help the child compensate for his particular deficits in the learning process, and at the same time, he continues to develop his learning strengths. The ultimate goal is for the child to be able to increase his academic skills as a result of the remedial help that is directed toward readiness requirements for academic achievement.

In the past, prior to the recognition of the particular sensory process needs of LD children, a child of normal intelligence who was unable to learn basic academic skills in reading and arithmetic was usually given special tutoring in the deficient skill per se. Today, the LD concept of special help means that remedial help will also be directed toward the learning processes that are fundamental underpinnings for acquiring the skills of reading, writing, or arithmetic. Ideally, such help should be offered to the child at the earliest possible time. To wait until the child has failed to acquire basic academic skills may well mean that the child will develop secondary emotional and behavioral problems.

The conceptual use of the multidimensional learning process model outlined in Fig. 5-1 immeasurably enhances communication of test results and consequent remedial plans to a teaching staff. For too long, teachers, and for that matter many professionals and lay persons, have thought of intellectual potential in terms of a single IQ score. Some persons even have the misconception that a child is born with an IQ. The IQ as a measure of the rate of development of a child's general intelligence is a valuable measure when correctly used and interpreted. This is particularly so if the intelligence test findings are combined with and interpreted in relation to a number of other test results that reveal developmental levels of visual-motor and linguistic processes. The learning disability movement has forced educators to look behind the meaning of single test scores and to analyze subtest measures on the basis of interest and intratest results of individual children.

Consequently, the psychological evaluation should seek to assess in depth all the facets of the child's learning process by means of the following: an individual assessment of intellectual functioning; the measured assessment of complex visual-perceptual-motor functioning; behavioral observations of the child in a variety of settings; and the assessment of the level of emotional maturity.

ASSESSMENT OF INTELLECTUAL FUNCTIONING

Frequently the LD child has wide scatter between varied measures of intelligence, suggesting a pattern of differences in the various processes required to perform the particular test items. A commonly used, individually administered intelligence test is the Wechsler Intelligence Scale for Children (WISC, 1949), which is used with children from 5 to 16 years of age. Children aged 4 years to 6 years six months can be given the Wechsler Preschool and Primary Scale of Intelligence (WPPSI, 1967). An advantage of the Wechsler as opposed to the Stanford-Binet test is that results offer a verbal IQ and a performance IQ, as well as a full-scale IQ. In contrast, the Stanford-Binet test results in only a single IQ, and any subtest analysis that differentiates visual-motor skills from auditory-verbal skills has to be done on a qualitative and scanning basis.

The verbal IQ of the WISC is the result of the scores of five or six subtests, all of which are heavily dependent on auditory input and verbal expressive ability. The performance IQ is based on five or six subtests, all of which are heavily dependent on visual input and motor expressive skills. LD children many times show wide discrepancies in their ability to pass these different tests. For example, a youngster may secure a verbal IQ of 140 (100 = average expectancy) and a performance IQ of 80, with a resulting full-scale IQ of 113. A glance at the latter single score tells us merely that the child is measuring in the above-average range, but knowledge of the other two scores tells us that the child is superior in verbal skills and very low average in performance skills. Such information is a clinical red flag, suggesting that further analysis of subtest measures is warranted. The psychologist must run more tests to analyze the total mosaic of the child's strengths and deficits.

There is much disagreement among psychologists as to the weight that should be placed on the meaning of test scatter on the WISC. There have been a number of attempts to establish a "brain damage" or "organic" pattern that will assure such a diagnosis, but no reliable pattern has been found. Nevertheless, the WISC is a well-standardized test and offers a good measure of various important areas of intellectual functioning in a way that no other instrument does. In relation to the analysis of learning process dysfunction, it is a vital adjunct to a full battery of visual-motor and linguistic measures. The meaning of the WISC subtest scatter in and of itself should not be overrated, for such scatter is merely suggestive of a need for further testing and investigation of measured deficits. It also suggests a need for looking into other underlying learning process dysfunctions that may have caused the low WISC subtest scores. For instance, when a child scores low on the object assembly test (a task that requires making a whole picture from parts), the following questions might be asked: Is the problem one of figure-ground difficulty? Is there a motor deficit? Is the child unable to perceive a whole that might be created from such parts? Or does the problem relate to errors in spatial orientation? The clinician then seeks the answers to these questions by examining the results of other tests that require the child to use similar processes. The WISC measures high-level cognitive skills and will not necessarily show a pattern of results that will indicate particular learning process dysfunctions. The same holds true for the WPPSI, which has proved to be a welcome addition to the field of testing young children. The test is similar in structure and scoring to the WISC. Tasks used in subtests require similar processes to those demanded by the WISC, but they are geared down to skills expected of younger children.

These measures thus give an idea of a child's language and performance skills. Should there be a major problem in language—in verbal skills—the psychologist might well run additional language tests or might refer the child for speech and language evaluations. Full discussion of the latter kind of diagnosis will be considered presently.

ASSESSMENT OF VISUAL-PERCEPTUAL-MOTOR FUNCTIONING

As already noted some items of the above intelligence tests require visual-motor abilities; for example, aspects of the performance tasks, such as the coding task, require fine eye-hand coordination and the ability to perceive visually presented symbols. The object assembly task requires that a child has mastered form constancy and has been able to separate figure from ground. These tests also have high-level cognitive aspects. Consequently, it is necessary to use some other measures that assess more directly a child's specific aptitude for developing skills in form constancy, figure-ground discrimination, spatial relations, fine eye-hand coordination, and position in space. There are a number of tests that have been devised with the evaluation of such skills in mind, such as the Marianne Frostig Developmental Test of Visual Perception, the Purdue Perceptual-Motor Survey (Roach and Kephart), and the Beery Developmental Test of Visual-Motor Integration.

The Frostig test has five subtests related to five areas: eye-hand coordination, figure-ground discrimination, form constancy assessment, position in space, and spatial relationships. These are reported to be five discrete tests of perception, but experience suggests that there may be considerable overlap among them. Normative data were improved with the second edition. There are no other instruments that tests these particular skills, and they are clinically helpful tests when joined with all other data.

A useful visual analysis test, easily administered, is the Columbia Mental Maturity Scale, devised by Burgemeister et al. This test measures a child's ability to perceive differences in forms, moving up to a high level of differences in concepts of things that go together. There is minimal motor ability required and no verbal expression needed.

Another measure of a child's level of form perception development, joined with a measure of eye-hand coordination, is to be found in the Beery test, which is easily administered in a standardized manner. The child is asked to copy a number of forms that become progressively difficult. Age level of ability is based on his performance up to the point of having three consecutive failures. The exactitude of the normative data and the truly developmental construction of the test are noteworthy.

The tasks set forth in the Purdue Perceptual-Motor Survey give still further indicants to help in evaluation. This survey encompasses the following areas of perceptual-motor development: balance and postural flexibility, body image and differentiation, perceptual-motor match, ocular control, and form perception. Evaluation is necessarily judgmental and can be very subjective. However, when the test is administered repeatedly by the same examiner, reliability of results can improve markedly. Again, though, these observations add another valuable dimension toward understanding the child who shows a wide range of visual-motor difficulties. The test also entails gross motor evaluation, which is not given consideration in any other tests.

As already noted there are a number of other measures, some dating from an early point in time, when Goldstein, as well as Strauss and Lehtinen, was concerned with the visual-motor problems of the brain-damaged persons with whom they worked. A full review of such tests can be found in Taylor or Burgemeister.

BEHAVIORAL OBSERVATION AND ASSESSMENT

A teacher's and parent's observations of a child over a period of time furnish essential information to the educational diagnosis. Many teachers have behavioral checklists that give some general guidelines for determining shifts that may have occurred over the time they have known a particular child. This information is helpful, but it is generally very global. It is even more significant for the teacher and parent to be able to consider the child's behavior pattern in relation to what might be expected for a particular chronological age. It should be recognized that the younger the child, the broader is the range of "normal" behavior. The high-risk child shows continuing deviancy in a number of dimensions, and this kind of deviancy can be assessed through home and school observation.

It is helpful for the teacher to have some knowledge of age norm yardsticks. An excellent measure, with age norms from 2 to 7 years, is available in Doll's Preschool Attainment Record, an observation checklist. This results in a summary eight-dimension profile related to physical, social, and intellectual development. The eight dimensions assessed are ambulation, manipulation, rapport, communication, responsibility, information, ideation, and creativity. This test provides a measurement of observed visual-motor, speech, and language behavior patterns as well as of observed social interaction. The resulting summary profile helps convey in a concrete manner to parents the range of skill development present in a particular child. Should verbal skills prove to be significantly deficient, there is an additional observation scale for the teacher to use—the Verbal Language Development Scale, by Mecham. This test measures additional aspects of verbal development from birth to 15 years of age.

Another normative scale that includes behavioral observations along with some easily administered visual-motor and language tasks is found in The Meeting Street School Screening Test (Hainesworth and Siqueland), with age norms from 5 to 7½ years of age. The immediate purpose of this scale is to give kindergarten teachers a simple way of screening children to determine whether more extensive evaluation is needed. The teacher or an intelligent lay person who knows the child well can make observations and administer the simple tasks; screening for a single child takes about 20 minutes. Again, these measured behavioral observations would be of considerable help in counseling a parent with respect to the range of behavior patterns and skills of a child. An additional purpose of the Meeting Street School Screening Test was to enable kindergarten teachers to have some accurate measurement of a child's development to help them make decisions about future school and grade placement.

A rapidly growing method of systematic measurement of behavior observation is being stimulated by professionals who are interested in behavior modification and whose theory and practices have stemmed from sociology and experimental psychology. This is a systematic way of assessing baseline measurements of observed behavior, followed by analysis of the stimulating circumstances. A treatment plan is then made to help modify the behavior of a student in terms of certain teacher-established goals. Behavior has been modified with respect to both cognitive and social behavior patterns. Baseline data on behavior patterns are collected over a period of time and followed by assessment of the behavioral and environmental components that maintain and modify the child's behavior.

The work of Lovitt with LD children is an example of focusing on objective, systematic, charted baseline behavior measurements, followed by investigation of these components of behavior: antecedent or stimulus event; movement or response behavior patterns of the child; and temporal arrangement or contingency systems involved in maintaining behavior. On the basis of these behavioral components, remediation plans are made and environmental changes effected to develop new behavior patterns. Basic to behavior modification theory is the reinforcement theory of learning derived from Skinner's work with animals. The principles have increasingly been applied to human learning. Recognition is given to the importance of positive reinforcement in promoting learning and to the failure of negative reinforcement in stimulating learning. A working knowledge of these consequences is of great importance to teacher-child relations as well as to parent-child relations. A clear and concrete explanation of basic behavior modification theory, appropriate for use with parents and teachers, is set forth by Wittes and Radin. The reader wishing a more thorough discussion of theory and practice is referred to Bijou and Baer.

ASSESSMENT OF LEVEL OF EMOTIONAL MATURITY

The LD child often has behavior patterns that may include one or more of the following: hyperactivity, emotional lability, problems in spatial orientation, distractibility and inattention, poor impulse control, and periodic daydreaming. The child who does not have a specific learning disability may also evidence similar behavior symptoms to an abnormal degree. The latter child would be said to have a primary emotional problem. The former, the LD child, would be said to have a secondary emotional disturbance, an overlay that is consequent to constitutional imbalance. Differential diagnosis in this regard is frequently very difficult to establish. In the instance of continuing emotional problems, the school and educational specialists will necessarily have to seek outside psychological and psychiatric help.

It is interesting in the history of seeking to help children who are unable to learn in school that, until the advent of the LD movement, the strong tendency of school guidance personnel was to immediately refer a bright child for psychiatric or psychological evaluation when he was unable to learn. The assumption was that there was some kind of "emotional block" that was impeding learning, and when outside psychological or psychiatric therapy removed the block, the child would then learn. In many instances the referral habit resulted in two worlds for the child, because there was poor communication or no communication between his teachers and his therapist. All too often the child experienced little increase in success in academic skills.

In the early 1960's the work of Cruickshank, who had been heavily influenced by Goldstein and had worked with Strauss, led to the increasing conviction among educators that, whether the child's behavior problems were consequent to constitutional deficits or emotional disturbance, the importance of the kind of classroom structure was great, and, probably, the learning requirements were the same. This issue is still far from settled, but the responsibility of educators and the importance of the teacher's role in helping both kinds of children are now well established. Furthermore, it is now apparent that many youngsters previously diagnosed as primarily emotionally disturbed had, instead, patterns of learning process disabilities that led to school failure and in turn to emotional problems.

A real danger, in this writer's opinion, now exists that children who are primarily emotionally disturbed will be misdiagnosed as LD children and not referred for psychotherapy or counseling. It should also be recognized that there are some LD children who may need some form of psychotherapy or counseling at some point in their lives. The children who have a flaw in processing outside stimuli, who readily find the world too much with them, are going to have more difficulty maintaining emotional equilibrium than those who do not have such a flaw.

Consequently, in any total psycho-educational diagnosis, particularly when the degree of emotional and behavioral disturbance is marked, there should be included a full clinical psychological battery of tests plus psychiatric evaluation. The clinical psychologist has skills in projective testing to help ascertain the level of emotional integration of a particular child. Traditionally, the Bender test, the Children's Apperception Test (CAT), the Thematic Apperception Test (TAT), and the Rorschach test have been used in this regard. These tests are not given by school guidance personnel but instead by clinical psychologists in private or clinic settings.

The clinical differentiation of the perceptually handicapped from the emotionally disturbed child is frequently difficult to establish. Sometimes, it is possible to make such a differential diagnosis only after observing and noting results over a period of time in an educational setting. For instance, consider a severly phobic child who initially evidences a defined cluster of subtest deficits in varied visual-motor processes. Such a child comes to mind who, after receiving instruction in a carefully structured situation and undergoing psychotherapy, proved to have superior measurements in all processes, auditory-verbal and visual-motor. The visual-motor deficits were no longer present. The learning profile of a child with a "specific learning disability" would not change so dramatically. Generally speaking, we have found that individual learning profiles of LD children remain the same in terms of patterns of strengths and weaknesses—that is, a child with lower measurements in visual-motor skills will always measure better in verbal skills and do less well in many performance tasks, or, vice versa, a child with comparatively low scores in verbal skills and high scores in visual-motor skills will always do less well in language than in performance tasks. Thus, the distinction between the emotionally disturbed nonlearning child and the LD child with secondary emotional disturbance is difficult and is frequently clarified only after a period of time. For instance, in the care of the aforementioned phobic child, one might hypothesize that the initial evidence of a significant perceptual deficit was his fear of looking, seeing, and revealing himself, rather than his inability to perceive.

In view of the frequent overlap among the emotionally disturbed and the learning-disabled groups, it is unfortunate that educational services for the two groups have been dichotomized by the structure of federal funding related to teacher training. The result has been the establishment of separate training sequences for teachers to work with both ED and LD children. Many states fund separate classrooms for ED and LD students. A few states, California for one, do not dichotomize, but instead have a broad category of children termed educationally handicapped. It is suggested that educators might think more realistically in terms of most learning-disabled children (types I and II learning disorders) as educationally handicapped, with only a small percentage actually classified as severely emotionally disturbed or as having a specific learning disability. The question of how the public educational system can best plan to meet the varying needs of all these youngsters has not been finally answered. Current theory and practices will be more fully discussed at the end of the chapter.

Language evaluation

The evaluation of language skills is an essential part of any diagnosis of learning disabilities. These linguistic abilities involve communicating and thinking in language symbols. Speech problems per se may not necessarily be present with linguistic disabilities; the presence of speech does not ensure the ability to communicate. Speech is the articulation of sounds and sound patterns, whereas language is the ability to communicate in a meaningful manner. It is possible for a child to have language and speech problems, speech problems alone, or language problems alone.

The importance of a child's level of language development is great, particularly in relation to making realistic and reliable estimates of his potential for academic achievement. There is a high correlation between vocabulary and language comprehension, and success in school subjects. The exact relationship between the development of verbal skills and early development in visual-motor skills is not known. A number of professionals (Barsch; Frostig; Getman and Kane; Kephart; and Strauss and Lehtinen) have placed great emphasis on perceptual-motor development as a necessary foundation for language development. In the LD movement considerable emphasis has been placed on remediation related to visual-motor development. Consequently, the LD child has frequently been linked with visual-motor problems, at times almost to the point of exclusion of concern about development of auditory-verbal skills. Our experience has been that many youngsters with learning disorders do have clusters of visual-motor deficits; however, many prove to have various combinations of auditory-verbal difficulties that frequently add up to major deficits in language. Such deficits can take varied forms in relation to receptive, associative, or expressive problems. Thus, in any psycho-educational evaluation it is imperative that careful and thorough evaluation be made of a child's language skills. There are a number of tests available to determine the level of verbal and nonverbal language abilities. This area of evaluation has been the bailiwick of speech and hearing professionals, with particular contributions made by Johnson and Myklebust. A full discussion of speech articulation testing, hearing testing, and language assessment is to be found in Myers and Hammill.

The Illinois Test of Psycholinguistic Abilities (ITPA) is a comprehensive test of children's language development. A child's scores, secured on the varied subtests of the ITPA, add another dimension to the scores secured on the WISC or WPPSI. The 1968 revised edition of the ITPA (Kirk et al.) consists of ten discrete subtests and two supplementary subtests. Six of the subtests measure aspects of the representational level of language, including two tests each of receptive, associative, and expressive language. The construction of these six subtests is such that three require predominant use of visual and visual-motor processes, and three require predominant use of auditory and auditory-verbal processes. The remaining subtests assess automatic functions, with two measuring sequential immediate memory, both visual and auditory. The other four tests assess varied aspects of auditory and visual closure. The intertest and intratest variability of a given child's performance on the ITPA gives the clinician further clues regarding the particular kind of process dysfunctions that may be present. This enables the clinician to hypothesize, on the basis of the learning model (Fig. 5-1), wherein the learning process disability(ies) of a child may lie, and consequently gives clues regarding the kind of remedial work needed to help the child compensate for his disabilities.

Additional language tests may be needed to further specify the cluster of process difficulties. For instance, the Peabody Picture Vocabulary Test (Dunn) gives information about a child's ability to identify objects and concepts on a nonverbal basis. The verbal subtests of the Stanford-Binet test or the WISC give further clues about the level of a child's language development.

The ITPA as a diagnostic and remedial model proved to be an instrument that gave educators a new approach to LD children. The importance of the test in this regard cannot be overestimated. The conceptualization resulted from Kirk's years of experience in helping educate exceptional children with a wide range of learning disorders. Kirk indicated in 1968 that there were three varieties of learning disorders: academic disorders, nonsymbolic disorders, and symbolic disorders. Just how these three kinds of learning disorders relate to one another is not known; a reading problem can be seen as an academic disorder, but what part of the reading difficulties may be due to nonsymbolic or symbolic disorders? The ITPA has subtests that measure both symbolic and nonsymbolic abilities. To date, the 1961 experimental edition has not yielded research results that allow for drawing conclusions regarding the relationship between school achievement and performance on the ITPA test. Thus, at the present time one could have no assurance when training a child in abilities represented by ITPA subtests that such training would enhance his ability to read. Nevertheless, the instrument has proved to be a valuable tool and has served as an important stimulus to educators to focus on personalized teaching—to give careful consideration in curriculum planning to individual differences present within any single classroom. And the remedial concept of looking at the underlying learning processes rather than just at the level of an academic skill has opened challenging avenues for future research. A recent impressive review of research possibilities is presented in a monograph by Chalfant and Scheffelin.

Academic achievement evaluation

In evaluation of academic achievement, the focus is on diagnosing quantitative and qualitative aspects of levels of achievement in basic skills: reading, writing, spelling, and arithmetic. In contrast to language evaluation, which deals with the input, association, and output of vocal symbols, academic evaluation is concerned with the input, association, and output of graphic symbols. Clinical experience indicates that there are those children who have very adequate oral language skills— that is, the ability to deal with vocal symbols—but when faced with graphic symbols, they experience various kinds of academic difficulties.

The exact relationship between oral and graphic language systems is not known. It would therefore be incorrect to generalize the test results from one system to another. Tests related to both systems are prerequisite to a complete educational diagnosis. Therefore, it is both necessary and appropriate to discuss the direct assessment of graphic symbol development by means of varied kinds of achievement tests of reading, writing, and arithmetic skills. As noted earlier, the school-age child with a specific learning disability has a significant lag in one or more basic school skills—there is a marked discrepancy between his measured intellectual potential and his level of functioning in one or more basic school skills. In the preschool child, specific learning disorders would be found in significant deviations of development in readiness skills, learning processes presumed to underlie future academic achievement.

The focus here will be on qualitative aspects of graphic skills that should be evaluated, rather than on an extensive discussion of achievement or diagnostic reading tests per se. A full review of the latter is available in Ashlock and Stephen. The academic testing of the school-age child is done through the administration of a battery of tests selected to evaluate his levels of functioning in basic skills. The testing of the preschool child involves the administration of diagnostic readiness tests, with results presumably indicating potential for reading, writing, and arithmetic. We say "presumably" because readiness tests have not proved to be valid predictors of a child's ability to learn to read. Pick, who has done extensive work in relation to basic perceptual processes required in the act of reading, feels that much additional basic research is needed in the area of selecting relevant reading predictors, because readiness tests as valid measures of reading potential do not exist. More often than not, the assumption is made that a high percentile score on a given readiness test ensures a child's readiness to read. The validity of this assumption has not been demonstrated.

The promise of discovering true predictors for determining the future academic success of young children may be realized in the intensive and extensive work of DeHirsch et al., who seek to develop a "predictive index" derived from researched parts of several tests. Again, the recently researchd and published Meeting Street School Screening Test (Hainesworth and Siqueland) may prove more valuable than readiness tests per se. In any event, the difficulty of assessing academic readiness in the young child is great. Nursery school and kindergarten teacher observations, plus the psychological and language evaluation of learning processes in individual high-risk preschoolers, need to be joined together to determine optimal educational planning for such children.

The psycho-educational diagnostician's particular interest in school achievement tests lies in the assessment of modality strengths and weaknesses on an input and output basis rather than in global grade level test scores. Overall grade level scores are important for in school administration. Also, such scores, when reviewed over a period of years from kindergarten to present grade placement, can furnish significant information about an LD child. However, within any single administration of an achievement battery, it is the profile of academic abilities that has particular diagnostic significance in relation to the goal of specific remediation.

There are six general areas involved in academic evaluation: (1) oral and silent reading ability, (2) oral and silent reading comprehension, (3) listening comprehension, (4) phonic and other word attack skills, (5) oral and written spelling ability, and (6) oral and written arithmetic ability.

The first five areas relate to aspects of academic achievement that are assessed in a battery of reading tests. Important work has been done in this regard through the years by professionals interested in developmental reading. As already noted, reading experts have long been concerned with helping children with learning disorders. Their testing and remedial expertise, together with the development of innovative concepts relating to learning processes, will hopefully result in additional answers for bright children who have severe reading problems of various kinds.

In a reading test battery the examiner is provided with estimates of a child's ability to respond to graphic symbols in terms of visual and auditory input, and vocal and motor output. This kind of qualitative analysis can give clues related to deficit modalities that could help determine the optimum teaching method for a particular child—a primarily phonic approach, a visual approach, or a multisensory approach.

The sixth area of evaluation concerns oral and written arithmetic. Inasmuch as achievement tests in arithmetic are all in written form, the examiner needs to use two forms of the same test, giving one orally and one on a written basis. Some youngsters handle number processes and concepts very well on an oral basis but cannot handle them at all in written form. Their problem might be one of visual perception, or it could be related to actual difficulties in eye-hand coordination, in which the act of writing is difficult. Further qualitative aspects to investigate relate to how the child handles computation and reasoning problems. Word problems should be given orally as well as in written form.

The examiner looks at these test results in terms of one mode of input against one mode of output. He seeks to answer such questions as the following: Does the child spell better on an oral or a written basis? Is reading comprehension better when someone reads to him or when he reads aloud or to himself? What is his level of comprehension when he reads to himself, as opposed to when someone is reading to him? Does the child write out a word better when it is given to him visually, or when it is spelled aloud to him? In this way the academic evaluation seeks information about the child's best modes of input and output in relation to manipulating graphic symbols as he is confronted with various kinds of reading, arithmetic, spelling, and writing tasks.

Further clues relating to a child's best modes of learning can be secured through informal kinds of testing of sound-letter and letter-sound associative abilities. The following combinations can be assessed:

1. *Auditory-vocal.* The sound is presented by the examiner, and the child responds with the name of the letter.
2. *Auditory-motor.* The sound of the letter is given, and the child is asked to write the letter.
3. *Visual-vocal.* The letter is shown to the child, and he verbally gives the name of the letter and the sound associated with it.
4. *Visual-motor.* The child observes the letter and then writes it after it has been withdrawn from sight.

All these diagnostic achievement data are combined with the findings from the psychological and language evaluations, resulting in a total profile of learning strengths and weaknesses for a particular child.

PSYCHO-EDUCATIONAL SYNTHESIS—A CHILD'S LEARNING PROFILE

The synthesis of all these evaluations leads to recommendations for curriculum planning and teaching methods that are believed to maximize the child's chances of compensating for learning process difficulties. The summary report should be made in such a manner that it is readily understood by educators and, above all, by the child's teacher. In addition, it is important for the parents of the child to come to understand the manner in which the child will best be able to learn. For instance, if a child has auditory discrimination problems, it is going to be difficult for him to retain and act on a series of verbal directions. The parents can help him by giving limited verbal directions and by using all the visual clues possible to ensure that the child knows what he is expected to do; this approach will also help build his memory skills.

Parent counseling in this regard needs to be concrete and specific. When true communication does occur, it is interesting to observe the insight gained by a parent, who may say, "And to think I just thought he was purposely tuning me out," or "I thought he was just too lazy or stupid to remember to do what I asked of him." Parents come to have realistic expectations through clarified knowledge of how the child best learns about the world around him, and they are thus able to help him compensate for areas of deficit. In the process of understanding the problem, they also enhance their relationship with the child as well as his own self-concept.

The learning profiles that emerge from these combined evaluations are many and complex, differing qualitatively and quantitatively for each child. Perhaps someday we will know enough about clusters of learning process difficulties to talk about particular kinds of learning disability profiles in a more specific way. For instance, in the type III disorder category, one might find input and output modality patterns that would be characteristic of severe reading, arithmetic, spelling, and writing problems. Type II disorder patterns would be characteristic of less severe academic difficulties, differing in quality and degree from type III. However, we are a long way from being able to talk in terms of a correlation between particular patterns and certain basic skill disorders. We are even farther from being able to make causal statements between particular deficits and basic skill disorders; for example, it cannot be said that children who have perceptual-motor problems will have reading problems. Professionals who draw unfounded conclusions of this kind are doing a great disservice to the learning disability movement.

Despite the present limitations in knowledge, the concept of diagnosing disabilities in learning processes on an input-association-output model is an important contribution to both regular and special education. It results in a different way of perceiving and working with a child who is unable to learn in school, giving a teacher a new way of approaching the child's learning difficulties. Too often in the past, schools have had the rule that remedial work is not done until after third grade, when the child has definitely proved that he cannot learn by regular curriculum methods. Remedial work then consisted of more of the same—more reading or more arithmetic. In contrast, LD theory causes a teacher to identify and help a child at an earlier point and to seek to understand underlying learning process difficulties, carrying out specific learning process remediation along with formal remedial work in the basic skill that is deficient.

Furthermore, the singling out of LD children has had far-reaching consequences in terms of federal and state legislation; the establishment of teacher training programs at universities, with certification in "Learning Disabilities"; the development of a national network of state and local parent groups under the National Association for Children with Learning Disabilities; and the development of private and public education facilities to meet the needs of LD children.

EDUCATIONAL PROGRAMS FOR CHILDREN WITH LEARNING DISABILITIES
A private-school program—Miriam School
BACKGROUND

Miriam School in Webster Groves, Missouri, a suburb of St. Louis, is a private nonprofit day school that has developed a pilot educational program to meet the needs of children with normal intellectual potential who have had significant learn-ing and/or emotional disorders in school. The goal is to enable youngsters to return to a regular school as rapidly as possible. The school is one of the main philanthro-pies of the Miriam Foundation, Inc., the philanthropic branch of Miriam No. 17, the local Lodge of the United Order of True Sisters, a national organization with headquarters in New York City. The philosophy of the Miriam Lodge is to initiate projects that meet unmet community needs and then to stimulate others to act to meet the needs.

In 1962 there were no public school programs in the greater St. Louis area for children of normal intelligence who were having difficulty in school due to learning disabilities and/or emotional disorders. Consequently the Miriam Lodge decided to start a pilot educational program that would serve such children.

The Miriam project that immediately preceded the 1962 project had been a school for retarded children, carried on since 1956. Public special education to meet the needs of the retarded child had developed rapidly, and it was for this reason that the Miriam School was able to turn its attention to the new program for children of normal intelligence. The years of experience with retarded children were an important asset and stimulus toward a better understanding of LD children. In diagnosing and educating retarded children, the staff had realized the many differences among retarded children; in some instances, children who had been diagnosed as retarded were discovered to be normal. The small, highly specialized classrooms at Miriam School had made it possible for some children who measured in the educable retarded range (by state law, the educable retarded range is between 48 and 78 IQ) to blossom forth and prove to have average or better-than-average intellectual potential. Such experiences had made the Miriam staff cognizant of dis-parate learning processes and of the extent of variability that might occur within a particular child.

As the Miriam School phased out the program for retarded children, the learn-ing disability movement was simultaneously developing more refined diagnostic techniques. The boom of LD curriculum development followed soon after. At the inception of the new program, Miriam School was most fortunate in securing consulting services from the University of Illinois' Institute for Research on Exceptional Children, headed by S. A. Kirk. Training in administration and re-medial use of the Illinois Test of Psycholinguistic Abilities was given to the Miriam staff through monthly consultation with Corinne Kass, Ph.D., assistant to Dr. Kirk. This opportunity opened the whole LD concept to the Miriam staff and stimulated the many developments in theory and practice that have fol-lowed.

SCHOOL STAFF

The director, a clinical psychologist, is assisted by a social worker who serves as parent consultant and liaison with community agencies. Special part-time educa-tional and psychiatric consultants meet on an alternating basis with the staff, which includes six classroom teachers, a speech and language therapist, a perceptual-motor teacher, and a physical education teacher.

An extensive volunteer training program makes available a corpe of well-qualified and supervised teacher-aides. Various other roles for volunteers develop as particular needs arise. During any one year the number of volunteers serving the children and staff will vary from 55 to 65. As the LD concept developed we came to have remedial volunteer teachers not only in arithmetic and reading but also in language, perceptual-motor work, memory work, and handwriting. A recent trend, as younger children have been admitted, has been to incorporate within the classroom curriculum all these vital learning areas, with special help offered to each classroom teacher by the speech and language therapist and the perceptual-motor teacher. A network of professional supervision of volunteer aides is carefully planned and scheduled.

The director of Miriam School and the Miriam School Board, a committee of Miriam Lodge, are fortunate in having the ongoing availability of counsel from an advisory committee composed of twelve professionals in the community. This committee is interdisciplinary in nature, with selection of disciplines determined by relevancy to the school program. Advisory committee members rotate off every three years, with provision for one repeat term at the discretion of the school director.

ENROLLMENT

INTAKE PROCESS. Referrals to the school are made by community agencies such as clinics, family agencies, and schools. Private practicing professionals also refer many youngsters. As the knowledge of the program has spread and our purposes have come to be understood by parents, there have been direct inquiries by parents. Application for enrollment is made by the parents. After application is made, all medical, psychological, and educational records are secured. The parents are interviewed by the Miriam social worker, and the child is interviewed by the director and the teachers in whose classrooms the child might be appropriately placed. They see the child both individually and in a group. The staff then meets with the school psychiatric consultant, jointly reviewing all the material about the child, the evaluations from outside sources, and the impressions received by members of the Miriam staff. After this conference the staff recommendations are conveyed to the parents by the school director.

ADMISSION CRITERIA. When the program began, children were admitted up through the age of 10 years. Since that time public school services have opened up for school-age children who have emotional and/or learning disorders. Consequently, Miriam School lowered the age of admission to 3 to 7 years. There are no restrictions as to race, color, or creed. A realistic scholarship program makes it possible for children of all socioeconomic levels to enroll. Strong parent-school relations are an integral part of the program, and all children live with their families.

It is hoped that all children admitted to the program have average or above-average intellectual abilities. Frequently this is difficult to determine in the young child, who may be hard to test due to either behavioral or developmental problems. A general rule of thumb is that the older the child at the time of admission, the more indicants of normal intelligence need to be evident. We endeavor not to admit children who give many indicants of retardation. We do admit many youngsters who have wide inconsistencies in learning abilities, with a range from retarded to superior. Many children also have achievement lags in skills expected of preschool and school-age children. Consequently, there is a broad range of academic and learning process disabilities among the children admitted to Miriam School.

There is also a broad range of emotional disorders represented in any single year's population at school, from the very passive, often daydreaming child, to the openly aggressive child. If a child is so severly disturbed that he appears to the staff to need a day-care or residential type of program, the family is referred to such resources. Should it be difficult to resolve the question of degree of disturbance, a decision may be made to recommend admission on a trial basis to determine if adjustment is possible for the child and for others in the class.

Past experience in having admitted preschool children who are too disturbed or too intellectually deficient led to the initiation of a special short-term observation program. This program is recommended to parents when there is a need for clarification with respect to appropriate educational placement, either at Miriam School or in another community facility. It involves having a child meet individually with a special teacher for three hourly sessions a week at Miriam School. Such sessions begin on a one-to-one basis and then may shift to classroom and varied group experiences, depending on the concerns the staff may have about a particular child, as well as the kind of relationship that develops between the child and the observation program teacher. The extent of the observation period is generally no longer than four weeks, after which time the director meets and counsels with the parents about educational planning for the child.

CLASSROOM STRUCTURE

TEACHING PHILOSOPHY. The Miriam staff does not believe that students, whether they have learning disability or emotionally derived problems, or both, can benefit from a laissez-faire or nonplanned environment. This holds true, in our experience, for children of school age as well as for those of preschool age. All youngsters who attend school, whatever their particular difficulty may be, need to respect the teacher and to understand and perceive her role as a teacher. In the history of education of emotionally disturbed youngsters, the role of the teacher has been perceived by some experts as that of a therapist. This thinking was largely developed in residential treatment centers, wherein the whole of the child's environment was spoken of as a therapeutic milieu. All too often in psychiatric settings the teacher has actually been perceived by staff members as low man on the totem pole. And many times the dictates of psychiatric treatment led to the development of a permissive classroom structure. Experience at Miriam School has convinced us that the more disordered the child, the more specific the expectations and curriculum planning have to be. And the role of the teacher has to be clearly that of a teacher. The problems involved in therapy are to be directed toward that channel. This distinction helps the child sort out his world and goes a long way toward rehabilitating him so that he is able to return to the regular classroom.

Many nursery school teachers would not agree with this philosophy of classroom structure in teaching preschool children. Again, though, experience at Miriam School has convinced us that the more deficient the young child is, whether the deficit be emotional, cognitive, or both, the more specific the program and curriculum planning should be. Furthermore, there is increasing evidence that adult-guided stimulation of preschool children, as opposed to unguided and self-guided exploratory learning, produces higher levels of learning and adjustment (Fowler). This is particularly true of the disordered child. For instance, we have found that the preschooler with visual-motor problems will avoid tasks that require visual-motor skills. The child with speech and language problems will not seek to participate in activities that require verbal skills. On the emotional side, the child with impulse control problems needs to have an outer structure that will help ensure controls and maximize the chance for development of self-control. The child who tends to withdraw from contact with the world around him should be intruded upon and expected to perform certain tasks. Thus, the teacher needs to plan guided and appropriate experiences to help in deficit areas, seeking to maximize success through the use of the child's strengths and making realistic demands for performance completion. This kind of teaching cannot be rigid, for the teacher must be sensitive to motivational and emotional shifts that occur in the child. The variability of these children is noteworthy, and the teacher needs to be tuned in to the wide range of differences that occur within a child and within the group. The resulting structure of the environment is reassuring to the disordered child.

CLASSROOM COMPOSITION. Classroom size ranges from six to no more than eight children. The composition of a particular class will determine whether a teacher asks for a volunteer teacher-aide, enabling her to have a pupil-teacher ration of one to three, or one to four. In a class of preschool children, classroom aides are always used. As a class is formed, enhancement of teaching and of group dynamics is sought through heterogeneous grouping.

Consequently, a given class may include children with an assortment of behavior patterns—for example, the withdrawn, daydreaming child; the aggressive, impulsive child; and the fearful child. Experience has led to the realization that children can help each other because of their behavior differences. Given an appropriate and well-timed structure, the aggressive child serves to stimulate the withdrawn child in a positive way. The fearful child stands a better chance of overcoming fears in a group that does not include all fearful youngsters. The child who has problems relating to people needs to have the experience of being with other children who relate warmly to people.

Any one class will also include children with a wide range of differences with respect to learning profiles. Some children will have auditory-verbal problems, some will have visual-motor deficits, and some will have cross-modality difficulties (deficits in varied aspects of both visual-motor and auditory-verbal processes). Here again, optimum placement is sought at the time of admission, with the teaching goal in mind of grouping children in a way that will maximize the teaching skills of the particular teacher. Thus careful consideration is given to both temperamental and intellectual factors in individual children as the decision is made to place a child in a particular classroom .

BEHAVIORAL SHAPING TECHNIQUES. As the teacher begins to work with a group of children, seeking to blend and relate to the many individual differences in the group, she must consciously and actively develop structure and shape behavior. A prime consideration in program planning relates to behavioral shaping; the classroom time schedule must allow for individual behavior patterns in the group. Important factors in the children to be considered are length of attention span, ability to control and inhibit impulses, ability to carry through learning tasks to completion, and ability to assume responsibility. The curriculum demands made on each child will vary according to his own particular performance level with respect to these factors.

The ultimate goal is to have a youngster develop self-control and enjoy the experience of being involved in learning for the sake of learning itself rather than for some external reward. The paths toward achieving this goal are as different as are the behavior patterns of the children. Many children have short attention spans and need guided experiences to increase their ability to focus. A number prefer not to interact with people, remaining aloof, distant, and self-involved. Some of the youngsters are receiving psychotherapy, and a number of children receive medication. The school works closely with outside professionals involved with the children and keeps them informed of intellectual and behavioral growth in the classroom. We find that all these children need a structured classroom experience, with behavioral expectancies clearly defined.

Consistency in discipline is important. Limits and established rules give external security as a child develops emotional and internal security. Praise for positive behavior guides the child in learning how to handle social relations. Negative behavior is ignored when it neither impedes the learning situation for the group nor proves too stimulating for the child initiating the behavior. When negative behavior has to be recognized and dealt with, Redl's concept of the life-space interview has proved to be helpful. This concept enables the teacher to deal directly with the behavior and help the child understand and experience the meaning of his behavior as it is perceived by others. The concept of the life-space interview can also be of benefit to the teacher in helping the child understand the meaning of all kinds of behavior. It enables the teacher to make maximal use of momentary life experiences as they relate to long-term goals of improved social behavior. Another approach to helping children understand their own feelings as well as the feelings of others is found in the human development program of Bessell and Palomares. This is a carefully programmed series of group experiences related to the areas of awareness, mastery, and social interaction. The program can be carried out by the classroom teacher as frequently as she is able to fit it into the curriculum. We have been impressed with the simplicity of this program, and with its effectiveness in relation to 4- to 6-year-old youngsters.

These behavioral shaping techniques are found to be useful with both school-age and preschool children. The younger the child, the more precise the structure needs to be. It is significant that many regular nursery schools do not operate on this premise. Thus the atypical preschooler in a regular nursery school often has a real struggle adjusting. Length of time is an important factor. Many nursery schools divide activities into 30- and 45-minute periods. At the Miriam preschool program, in the initial phase of program planning, the day may have to be broken up into 10-minute sequenced intervals, alternating activities that require full group participation with periods of free play, when children seek activities of their own choosing. The concept of free play and self-directed activities has been an essential belief in regular nursery school and kindergarten programs for many years. It is our experience that complete freedom of choice often places a burden on the child who lacks emotional equilibrium. Free play for such youngsters may further individual pathology. For instance, it affords a chance for the child who withdraws to withdraw even farther. The child who tends to perseverate may become obsessively repetitive. The impulse-ridden youngster may become overstimulated. Consequently, free play periods frequently need guidance. In the instance of school-age children, length of recess periods and opportunities for free choice in classroom activity are determined by a particular group's tolerance for such freedom.

As behavior patterns of the group meld and the children become participating members, it is very informative to make use of sociometrics. A child's selection of another child with whom he would like to work or play gives valuable clues regarding optimum ways of breaking up the group so that the teacher can work with a few children while the aide works with others. It is also possible to team children together so that they help each other, both emotionally and intellectually. Proper grouping can allow a child to use his strengths to help the weaknesses of a classmate. As the group becomes cohesive, and the time span for activities lengthens, children remain integrated and involved for longer periods and become able to make valuable and constructive use of free time as well as becoming highly motivated for formal learning tasks.

CURRICULUM PLANNING

TEACHING PROCEDURES—BACKGROUND. As a small private school, Miriam has been able to be eclectic in selecting varied assortments of teaching procedures that have been developed by the many disciplines interested in the child who is disabled in learning. These procedures relate to teaching basic academic skills—reading, writing, and arithmetic. They also have to do with specialized methods concerned with preacademic training. These specialized approaches have been developed in direct relation to helping LD children compensate for various constellations of learning process deficits. This summary discussion will present an overview of some of the specialized approaches that have been developed.

In view of the many kinds of handicaps represented in the LD population, it is not surprising that many disciplines have come to have theories about educational procedures to be used. Some of these procedures were initially used with deaf children, some with blind children, some with children labeled dyslexic, aphasic, brain-damaged, or language-disordered, and some with retarded children. The label connected to the child for which the procedure was initially designed need not limit the usefulness of the procedure for children with other handicapping conditions. In this regard it is interesting to reflect on how the exciting methods that Maria Montessori used to stimulate deprived, retarded children in 1912 are today being used with a broad span of children, including bright, socially advantaged children. Many of her theories and sensory-motor experiences have been incorporated into preschool and special education programs.

For clarity of discussion, we will consider the varied educational procedures in terms of the primary sensory orientation emphasized by the particular procedure. Detailed discussions of these procedures are available in Myers and Hammill, and in McCarthy and McCarthy. Focus will be on four categories of educational systems: perceptual-motor systems, a neurophysiological system, language development systems, and multisensory systems.

Perceptual-motor systems. There have been many professionals concerned with LD children who have placed marked emphasis on special perceptual-motor training as a prerequisite to improving learning skills. Many of these techniques are similar to those used in readiness programs in most kindergartens. Each of the theorists has developed an instructional theory with respect to the use of these techniques on a developmental basis. The assumption is often made that when the child has achieved visual-motor skills expected at his age level, he can then move ahead and learn to read by the usual teaching methods. There is a wide range of literature in this regard, with primary contributors being Barsch, Friedus, Frostig, Getman and Kane, and Kephart. These techniques cover a range of developmental tasks related to fine and gross visual-motor development, including figure-ground perception, form constancy, spatial relations, visual sequencing, etc. Of the authors listed, Frostig and Kephart are the only two who have structured their theories and procedures around a series of tests used for diagnostic and evaluative purposes.

A neurophysiological system. Delacato has developed and written extensively about his theory of neurological disorganization as being the underlying cause of learning disabilities. He perceives his visual-motor development procedures as being a method of treating the nervous system in such a way that the child moves developmentally through missed stages of neurological development.

These procedures and his claims of diagnosing specific neurological impairments in relation to specific academic skill deficits have resulted in wide controversy and discussion. The controversy revolves around his assumption that it is possible to reorganize a child's nervous system by putting the child through specific motor training. Educators are in no position to make such statements. It is important for special educators to have full knowledge of Delacato's theory because many parents of handicapped children have become involved with the theory and then have come in direct conflict with the school. Delacato holds that at certain periods and for certain lengths of time, handicapped children should be held out of school and systematically given cross-patterning exercises at home. This conflict can place the school counseling personnel and the teacher in a difficult position with a child's family. Delacato maintains there is need for stringent research to prove the validity of his position.

Language development systems. Professionals who have been primarily concerned with language-impaired children have contributed a great deal with respect to both theory and actual teaching procedures used to aid in the development of auditory-verbal skills. Myklebust, Johnson, and McGinnis developed extensive procedures, with original interest being stimulated by their work with children having severe hearing impairments. Orton was stimulated to develop language teaching procedures consequent to his particular interest in children having severe reading problems. Inherent in a broad understanding of language development is the recognition that perceptual-motor procedures and language development procedures need to be combined in planning for a total program to meet the needs of LD children. Consequently, teachers working in special education do well to be knowledgeable in all procedures, because with any given child all procedures may be used at one time or another. During the initial focus on LD children, primary interest was in visual-motor procedures. Within recent years educators have recognized the tremendous importance of incorporating techniques and establishing goals that also emphasize the development of auditory-verbal skills.

Multisensory systems. A multisensory approach places emphasis on the use of kinesthetic and tactile modalities, as well as auditory and visual channels, to enhance learning. Fernald evolved a systematic way of teaching learning-disabled children. She found that children with particular problems in reading were helped through initial exercises using tactile and kinesthetic senses, leading to more and more dependence on auditory and visual modalities. Others who have developed multisensory theories and procedures are Ayres, Cruickshank et al., and Strauss and Lehtinen.

The development of all these educational theories and practices has led to the publishing of many kinds of teaching materials, some of them directly related to a particular theory, and others generated by the LD concept of relating teaching procedures directly to individual strengths and deficits. The result today is the availability of a wide assortment of sequentially planned programs concerned with varied aspects of visual-motor and auditory-verbal skills.

The danger inherent in the "cookbook" nature of some of the materials is the possibility that the teacher may feel impelled to follow all lesson directions and lose sight of the child. When carefully selected and properly used, such materials offer teachers many imaginative and developmentally planned teaching aids. For optimum use, it is essential for the teacher to have developed a hypothesis about a particular child's learning strengths and weaknesses, and then to plan a specific program of tasks, both academic and preacademic, that will enable the child to compensate for his weaknesses and at the same time enhance his strengths.

ANALYSIS OF LEARNING PROFILES—DEVELOPMENT OF CURRICULUM GUIDELINES. The selection of teaching tasks and procedures at Miriam School is aided by the diagnostic testing process. Miriam students, at the time of admission, have generally had a number of psychological tests. Additional tests are subsequently run, and the subtest scatter of each child is analyzed. The learning profiles of all students are analyzed on the basis of subtest measures of the Wechsler Intelligence Scale for Children (WISC) or the Wechsler Preschool and Primary Scale of Intelligence (WPPSI), the Illinois Test of Psycholinguistic Abilities (ITPA), the Purdue Perceptual-Motor Survey, the Peabody Picture Vocabulary Test, the Beery Developmental Test of Visual-Motor Integration, the Marianne Frostig Developmental Test of Visual Perception, and the Columbia Mental Maturity Scale. Additional important information is gained through speech and hearing tests run at the school and vision tests given by outside professionals at the time of admission.

The diagnostic clinical synthesis of these test results gives knowledge of each child's strengths and weaknesses in sensory-motor skills. A further synthesis is made of the six to eight individual patterns of learning abilities in each classroom, resulting in a total learning profile that informs the teacher of significant learning strengths and weaknesses present in the class as a whole. This knowledge then enables the teacher to plan learning process and academic tasks that will make maximum use of strengths and compensate for both individual and group deficits.

The individual learning profiles are many and varied. Some youngsters measure in the average or above-average range on subtests that require visual-motor skills but measure below average on subtests that require auditory and verbal skills. The profile of such a child is illustrated in Fig. 5-2. The graphed scores represent measures of ability to receive information about the world; to think about and associate with respect to such information; to remember on both an immediate and a delayed basis; and to express meaning through gestural, written, and verbal means. This particular profile, of a child whose chronological age (CA) was 7 years 3 months, shows average to well above average visual and visual-motor skills, as measured on the WISC, ITPA, Frostig, and Beery tests, with a range from 7 years 4 months through 10 years 6 months. In contrast, measured auditory-verbal skills were significantly deficient, ranging from 3 years 6 months to 5 years 6 months.

In Fig. 5-3 a reverse type of learning profile is illustrated graphically. This is a profile based on a CA of 7 years 6 months, with average to above-average measurements in tasks that require auditory and auditory-verbal skills. In contrast,

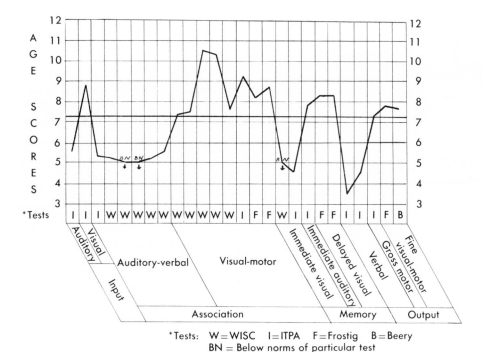

*Tests: W=WISC   I=ITPA   F=Frostig   B=Beery
BN = Below norms of particular test

FIG. 5-2. Learning profile with visual-motor strengths and auditory-verbal weaknesses.

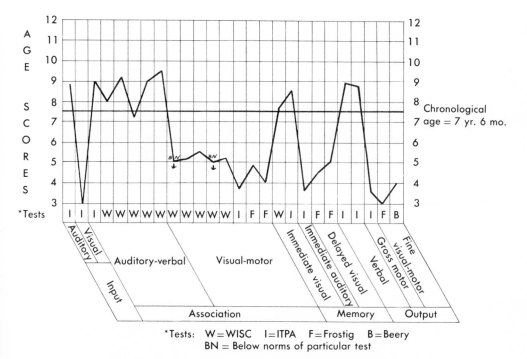

*Tests: W=WISC   I=ITPA   F=Frostig   B=Beery
BN = Below norms of particular test

FIG. 5-3. Learning profile with auditory-verbal strengths and visual-motor weaknesses.

the significantly low measures in this profile are in tasks requiring visual and visual-motor skills of various kinds. The range of visual-motor measures is from 3 years to 5 years 6 months; the range of auditory-verbal measures is from 7 years 3 months to 9 years 6 months.

Each class of youngsters includes an assortment of individual learning profiles. The group learning profile is a composite of the profiles of the individual members. Most individual learning profiles are not as clearly dichotomized with respect to visual-motor and auditory-verbal patterns as noted in the above illustrations. However, widespread scatter is typical of the LD child, and it is not uncommon for the scatter of low scores to occur in both visual-motor and auditory-verbal subtests. Such patterning may be considered to be that of a youngster with cross modality problems.

TEACHING TO INDIVIDUAL DIFFERENCES

Group teaching—school-age children. For the sake of both clarity and brevity we will present a classroom of six children who had remarkably homogeneous learning profiles; most classes find wider differences in individual learning patterns.

MRS. FINLEY'S CLASS   November, 1963

Student	CA	MA	IQ	Learning assessment		Achievement test October, 1963	Previous school experience
				Strengths	Weaknesses		
1	8-0	7-8	94 (S-B)		Visual association Visual memory Visual-motor	Mental readiness Reading= High normal Numbers= Average	Kindergarten and first grade in regular parochial school
		6-4	77 (WISC)	Motor expression Auditory-visual association Auditory association	Auditory memory Vocal ability Spatial concepts Short attention span Great hyperactivity		
2	7-5	5-10	77 (S-B)	Visual association Visual memory Auditory-visual association Auditory memory Vocal ability Spatial concepts Good attention span Hyperactivity diminishing	Visual-motor Motor expression Auditory association	Mental achievement Primary I Reading= Grade 1.6 Numbers= Grade 2.0	Public school kindergarten Miriam retarded program Miriam normal program
3	6-8	6-9	101 (WISC) V=96 P=106	Visual association Auditory-visual association Auditory association Auditory memory Vocal ability Spatial concepts	Visual memory Visual-motor Motor expression Short attention span and hyperactivity	Mental readiness Reading= Average Numbers= Superior	Private nursery school

A

FIG. 5-4. Learning profiles of special class of LD school-age children.

However, there were still many qualitative differences present, as noted in the summary chart in Fig. 5-4. The age range of these six youngsters at the start of the school year was from 6 years 3 months to 7 years 10 months. Mental ages, as measured by either a WISC or a Stanford-Binet test, ranged from 5 years 3 months to 7 years 10 months. Only one of the students was a girl. All but one child had previous school experience in nursery and kindergarten settings, private and public. One child had had experience in a parochial first grade.

A careful admission process had evaluated these children as having sufficient potential that they might at some time be able to fit into more normal classrooms. It was further judged at the time of admission that their learning and behavioral difficulties were severe enough to necessitate a special approach. Hyperactivity and short attention span were part of the symptomatology of four children out of six. The remaining two had the problem of withdrawal and consequent inattention. One of the latter (child 6 on the chart) was a seriously disordered child who had severe problems in relating to reality.

Of the six children, five were at a readiness point in learning. The sixth child

MRS. FINLEY'S CLASS   November, 1963

Student	CA	MA	IQ	Learning assessment		Achievement test October, 1963	Previous school experience
				Strengths	Weaknesses		
4	6-11	6-8	96 (WISC) V=97 P=94	Visual association Auditory-visual association Auditory association Auditory memory Vocal expression Fair attention span No hyperactivity	Visual memory Visual motor Motor expression Spatial concepts	Mental readiness Reading=High normal Numbers=High normal	Public school kindergarten
5	6-5	5-3	80 (S-B) (Inc.)	Auditory-visual (?) Auditory association (?) Vocal ability	Visual association Visual memory Visual-motor Motor expression Auditory memory Spatial concepts (?) Very short attention span Hyperactivity and stubborn behavior	Unable to test fully	Private nursery schools
6	7-9	?	?	Visual association Visual-motor (?) Motor expression Auditory memory	Visual memory (?) Auditory association (?) Vocal ability (?) Spatial concepts (?) Variable attention Reality problems	Not testable	Private nursery school

B

Fɪɢ. 5-4, cont'd. For legend see opposite page.

(child 2 on chart), who had come through the Miriam School program for re-tarded children, was already achieving all skills at a first grade level. He was the only child whose primary strengths were in visual areas, with major weaknesses in auditory and verbal channels. The other five children had strengths in auditory and verbal channels, and weaknesses in visual and motor areas.

Child 6 was difficult to test, and test results were very unreliable. All the other children had been tested on a full battery of tests: WISC; ITPA; Marianne Frostig Developmental Test of Visual Perception; Peabody Picture Vocabulary Test; Columbia Mental Maturity Scale; standard tests of achievement; and speech and hearing tests. All children were discussed by the staff in terms of classroom and individual approaches. The theory in planning classroom work for the school-age child is to make major use of sensory strengths and to plan individual compensatory work for sensory deficits. The individual work is sometimes carried on in the classroom and sometimes carried on outside. Both volunteer aides and other students help with such individual work. The single child with language problems (child 2) also worked individually with the language therapist.

The first month of school might be termed a conditioning process for a class. In this particular group, the attention span at the initial point was limited to 5-minute intervals. The teacher's goal at first was to achieve a 5-minute period in which all the children would be focusing. Group activity at desks began with the use of the tactile sense, the identification of forms by feeling, sorting, and tracing. Then activities were directed toward matching objects of the same shape. The remainder of the time, at this early period, was spent in rhythm activity, role play-ing of different animals and situations, and story time. All children also participated in the regular physical education program.

As attention span lengthened and the group became coordinated, much audi-tory work was conducted, with emphasis on rhyming. It was decided that a phonic approach to learning reading would be used for all five of the children who had not begun to read. This decision was based on the knowledge that the auditory channel was a strong one for all of them. By the end of October a sound chart was introduced, accompanied by pictures. A set of cards matching the letter and picture combinations on the chart was made. The letter was on one side of the chart and the picture on the other. Matching the cards to the chart, thus providing both auditory and visual stimulation, was a process that was initiated slowly and for increasingly longer periods each day.

Number concepts were introduced at about the same time and manipulated in such terms as large, small, and equal. The Stern blocks (1954) were used to ini-tiate the learning of number concepts. These blocks proved ideal because they are large, the different quantities are of differing colors, and the children related readily to tactile use of the blocks. No actual numbers were connected with any of the blocks. Learning, instead, came through matching like blocks, noticing blocks that did not match, and feeling the scored parts that made up the whole of an-other block.

Meanwhile, role playing and rhythm work continued, and gradually the daily schedule began to shape up. Longer and longer spans of time were spent on segments of readiness work. The homogeneity of sensory deficits in the group was not accompanied by homogeneity of behavior patterns. The range of behavior patterns was from the extremely withdrawn child (6), who often drifted off into fantasy, to the child (5) who was extremely negativistic and subject to readily aroused temper outbursts. The behavioral shaping of each child is done gradually and with specific goals and expectations in mind. Acknowledged limits and expectations were eventually accepted by all six children. However, the fantasy-ridden child (6), intermittently regressed and would not be "with it."

Finally, just about Thanksgiving time, formal reading was begun and a strongly phonic approach was used. Gradually the group built up to working at reading skills for as long as an hour at a time. Number work also progressed well and workbooks were introduced. Writing was difficult for most youngsters and progressed very slowly. The tactile method of feeling a letter, then tracing it, and then writing it was attempted, with limited success as first. Greater focus was on the underpinnings of writing, with much work on copying forms and encouraging fine motor development. Eventually cursive writing was introduced. Many youngsters with fine eye-hand deficits find it easier to write cursively. It has more flow and does not require stopping and starting individual letters, as required in manuscript writing.

Individual remedial programs for all children except child 6 were based on weaknesses measured by the ITPA and the Frostig test. This work also included gross visual-motor work relating to body image and awareness. Child 6 was not worked with outside the classroom, for it was believed that he needed the continual reassurance of being in one place and the stability of relating to a single teacher.

Thus it is that a teacher works with a group of significantly atypical children and plans specifically to meet individual learning process needs, while at the same time gearing the group to move ahead to achieve basic academic skills. As the children begin to cope and deal with learning tasks, the teacher then pushes toward more and more independence and makes appropriate academic demands.

Group teaching—preschool children. In planning for preschool children the process of analyzing individual and group learning profiles is carried out in a manner similar to that employed for school-age children. The same battery of tests (with the WPPSI used instead of the WISC) is used for the determination of individual and group deficit and strength patterns. The preschool years are an ideal time to identify deviant growth patterns and then seek to help maximize a child's intellectual potential through planned sequencing of tasks directed toward stimulating specific kinds of learning processes. The tasks are of the kind that interest all young children and are a part of the activities of all nursery schools and kindergartens. A major difference in the Miriam teaching philosophy from that of many nursery teachers is that children are expected to do certain things at certain times, and completion is expected of certain tasks, relating to both learning strengths and weaknesses. How specific the demands are will of course depend on the child's level of ability and tolerance for perseverance. Experience indicates that the pleasure of learning and of completing a task, joined with developing self-control, leads to the ability to create, to imagine, and to make decisions. A sample preschool classroom schedule, designed to meet the needs of six children—two girls and four boys—is presented in the following outline:

NOVEMBER 7, THURSDAY CLASSROOM SCHEDULE

11:45 to 12:00 Beginning quiet time activity

> As children enter they take off wraps, go to the round table, and start on quiet time activity, which on Thursdays is always working on puzzles.

12:00 to 12:20 Language work

TEACHER	VOLUNTEER AIDE
Charles Joe Jim	Mary Lee John
Ginn, Kit A, Language—Building Pre-Reading Skills, Review animal mothers and babies. Start Lesson C, p. 149, Real and Make-Believe	Peabody Language Development Kit, Level No. 1, 1965, Lesson No. 50, p. 62, Nos. 2 and 3

12:20 to 12:40 Free time—two choices to be offered to each child

> Aide—If Jim becomes too keyed up or aggressive, step in and enter into play situation to tone him down. If Joe moves off into dreamworld, make demands on him, involve him in task, giving him choices.

12:40 to 1:00 Group language work

> Peabody, Level P, Lesson No. 7, p. 12

1:00 to 1:20 Free time, followed by cleaning up of materials used in two free-play periods—for example, if large-block play begun earlier, then large blocks restacked by end of this second free time.

1:20 to 1:40 Visual-motor work

TEACHER	VOLUNTEER AIDE
Block design patterns with entire group. John, Mary, and Lee: low level; Jim, Joe, and Charles: high level	Gross motor, balance, and spatial relations, with Mary, Lee, and John taken out of group individually for 5-minute periods

1:40 to 2:00 Recess

2:00 to 2:30 Juice, rest, story

The learning process handicaps in the class included a child with a severe speech problem, one with a cross modality problem, and four youngsters with assorted visual-motor deficits. Emotional problems affected two children who had difficulty relating to both adults and peers, a child who was readily overwhelmed by fear, and two children who had problems controlling impulses.

Of particular note in the classroom schedule are the following: the small segments of time; the regularity of expectations from the moment the child enters the classroom; the flexible use of the aide; the sorting of learning groups according to specific learning process needs; the specificity of approach to individual developmental levels, even when the group as a whole is working together; and the expectancy of task involvement and completion.

As the group gains in cohesiveness and individual strength, the schedule is changed, allowing for greater learning expectations from individual children and leading to more free time—more opportunities to make independent decisions and choices by those children who prove to be able to cope with such responsibilities. In this particular group, four children have now returned to regular school, with all achieving well in academic skills. One child proved to have a specific learning disability and to be qualified for a public school special LD class. The single remaining child proved to be so disordered as to need residential care. Miriam School will follow with interest the progress of these youngsters. A regular yearly follow up questionnaire is sent to both parents and teachers of all children who have left Miriam School.

Individual programming in a type III LD—severe handwriting deficit. This is a case report of a girl who was an early reader (by age 3 years) despite severe problems in visual-motor areas, both gross and fine. She was an only child of older parents. The early medical history included problems of breathing at birth, followed by convulsive seizures at varied intervals. The seizures were brought under control by 4 years of age through medication. Her most severe developmental lag was in the area of fine eye-hand coordination, and there was also a significant lag in gross motor development. Her right side was considerably weaker than the left. She also experienced difficulties in balance, spatial relations, and depth perception. Visual acuity was normal after correction for myopia with glasses. Her body build was wiry, and she was significantly smaller in size than other children of her age.

Social and emotional development were also lagging. At the time she entered Miriam School, at 6 years 2 months of age, her self-awareness was markedly deficient, and she had little interaction with peers. She was able to relate to adults and was dependent on them. She was a very verbal child and had an automaton quality in her manner of expression. Prior school experience had included attendance at a regular public school kindergarten and a month in first grade. Social problems developed in relation to peers, as she proved to have minimal ability to relate to other children. She would either be extremely aggressive or withdraw. The marked visual-motor problems meant that she was unable to handle many classroom tasks. When asked to draw, she would uncontrollably scribble. She also had difficulty finding her way around and readily would become confused about where she was when out of the classroom. The public school had recommended evaluation, and referral was made to Miriam School. Base-line testing at

Student: S. C.   Birth date: 7-3-61

WISC: 9-67   V IQ=104   P IQ=65   FS IQ=84
        6-69   V IQ=124   P IQ=82   FS IQ=104

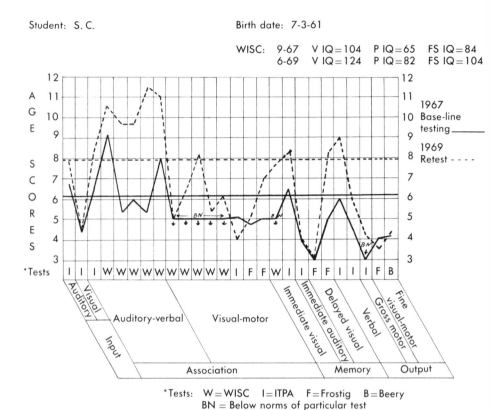

*Tests: W=WISC I=ITPA F=Frostig B=Beery
         BN = Below norms of particular test

FIG. 5-5. Profile of child with type III learning disability—severe handwriting deficits and spatial problems.

the time of the initial evaluation, when she was 6 years 2 months of age, is shown in Fig. 5-5. Her level of functioning in auditory-verbal skills ranged from a low of 4 years, 4 months in immediate auditory memory to a high of 9 years 2 months in general information. Vocabulary measured at the 8-year level. Most tasks requiring verbal skills were in the average range. In contrast, all tasks requiring visual-perceptual-motor skills were markedly deficient. The 39-point discrepancy on the WISC between the verbal IQ of 104 and the performance IQ of 65 was noteworthy. The range of functioning levels on visual-motor tasks was from two to three years below chronological age expectancy. The results of this base-line testing could only be considered an estimate of the visual-motor problem, inasmuch as norms at the lower levels of the tests, particularly on the WISC (which bases at 5 years), are not valid. In any event, it was apparent that this youngster needed major help in the areas of both gross and fine visual-motor coordination.

She was enrolled in a classroom of seven children. Her ability to read was remarkable, and her achievement in this regard continued. Number concepts were limited, although she did know number combinations to ten on a rote basis. A specialized program was carried out with respect to gross motor work, including much initial focus on body awareness, a sense of space, and understanding and experiencing right and left. Her deficits in these areas were marked. Concomitantly, work was also directed toward helping fine eye-hand and visual patterning deficits. Initial work related to tracing and feeling forms. Block pattern designs were kept simple and at a concrete level. Strengthening exercises for both her left and right hands were programmed, with the left side proving to be much stronger than the right. In doing all these tasks, her own verbal reinforcement of what she did was urged; for example, as she was walking a square, she would say, "I walk on this side, here is a corner I go around, here is another side," etc. The theory was to use the verbal strengths, joined with visual-motor experience, to enhance her awareness of the world around her, the objects in it, and her relationship to them. She was unable to crawl in a cross pattern, handling crawling in a froglike manner. Much work was done in motoric cross patterning that aimed at developing her motor kinesthetic sense of feel for patterned movement.

During her two years at Miriam School, programming continued in both the fine and gross visual-motor areas, with many program ideas based on the Frostig, Roach and Kephart, and Getman and Kane systems of perceptual-motor training. During the course of time it was interesting to note a diminishing of her robotlike quality as she came to be able to express feelings and emotions and began to emerge as a person. She continued to relate better to adults than to children but showed some beginnings of peer interaction.

In academic work she proceeded in reading but indicated some difficulty when inferences were required. Much of her verbal behavior was stereotyped. Number concepts began to develop in a manner that could not have been predicted on the basis of her marked difficulties in spatial concepts. By the time she left Miriam School at the age of 8 years, she had a good grasp of math concepts at a third grade level. At the time she was achieving in all academic skills at her expectancy level or above for her chronological age, except in writing. Progress in this skill continued to be slow. It was decided that, in addition to working directly on strengthening eye-hand control through pencil-and-paper work, it would be advisable for her to begin to learn typing. To this end, a typing program was developed that involved the use of the entire left hand and one finger on the right hand. She enjoyed this work, and at the time she left Miriam School, the family was seeking to continue her typing program.

A retest of all previously administered base-line tests was made at the point of leaving Miriam School, at CA of 8 years. Results are graphically given in Fig. 5-5. These measurements indicate that there is no question that she made significant gains in verbal skills and some gains in visual-motor areas. Her WISC verbal IQ shifted upward from 104 to 124, and her performance IQ from 65 to 82. In consequence, the full-scale IQ changed from 84 to 104. Two significant visual-motor subtest gains are found in the Frostig subtests of form constancy (a shift from 5 years to 8 years 3 months) and also in the WISC block design task (from below the 5-year norms of the test to 7 years 11 months). However, the other deficient areas continued to be present, with particularly low scores in eye-hand coordination (the Frostig subtest measured at 3 years 6 months), and her Beery perceptual age quotient simultaneously measured at 4 years 4 months.

Consequently, the learning profile remained essentially the same with respect to the degree of disparity between auditory-verbal strengths and visual-motor deficits. There was significant shift upward in verbal abilities, suggesting average to above-average strengths. Some compensation had occurred in spatial perception. However, the eye-hand deficit continued to be of such severity by age 8 that it was highly questionable how well she would be able to compensate for this handicap, which appeared to be both perceptual and motoric in nature. She also continued to need much support and direction in changing to new surroundings and meeting new expectations, problems that might be related to her continuing spatial difficulties. The pervasive nature of these continuing handicaps are strong indicants of the presence of a type III learning disorder, a disorder of such degree that this youngster will need the help of a special small classroom for some time to come.

At the conclusion of two years at Miriam School, referral was made to the special education district, where she was accepted in the program for neurologically handicapped children, which serves many youngsters with normal intellectual potential but varying kinds of physical impairment. The goal will be to have her return to the regular public school classroom if and whenever possible.

Individual programming in a type III LD—severe reading problem. This case report describes a boy who enrolled in Miriam School at 8 years 3 months of age, at which time he was unable to read and had no grasp of number concepts, despite a year of placement in a special class. Additional previous school experience had included kindergarten and first grade in a public school. In kindergarten he was described as a "naughty" boy who would fall off his chair for no reason. He was hyperactive, had a short attention span, and daydreamed a good deal of the time. He was promoted to first grade, where the same behavior continued and he proved to be unable to learn any symbols as they were presented to him on paper.

In reviewing developmental information, one sees nothing remarkable. Motor development was on the early side, and verbal behavior was also somewhat advanced for his age. A single illness, caused by tonsillitis, occurred when he was 2 years old, and at that time he suffered a temperature of 106° for two days. Otherwise, health was generally good. His mother noted that she had no difficulties during pregnancy but that she experienced extended hard labor at the time of birth. He is the only boy in the family, and he has two older sisters. One is deaf (the mother had rubella during pregnancy), and the other is proving to be a slow learner.

By the end of first grade the family became concerned and sought neurological evaluation, where findings were inconclusive. Medication was initiated and there was a marked decrease in hyperactivity. Admission to a child guidance clinic's special classroom was sought, with consequent full psychiatric and psychological evaluation. Concomitant with admission to the clinic classroom, supportive psychotherapy was initiated, with casework for the mother as well as for the father, at times when he would be home from regular Army duty out of the country.

His teacher in the special classroom had found him to be no behavior problem. Other children liked him, and he proved to be a leader. She had worked with him on phonic skills and also on number concepts and believed that at the time of his referral to Miriam School, he had made some progress. In actuality, his Miriam teacher discovered that he would gain a degree of ability to recognize some words and some numbers, and then lose all of his knowledge. From time to time in the first year and a half at Miriam School, all previous knowledge of written symbols would be lost from one day to the next. Consideration was repeatedly given as to whether these blockings might be emotionally derived. The psychiatric evaluation perceived the behavioral disorder as a reaction to his inability to learn. Miriam School's experience with him through the past three years appears to con-

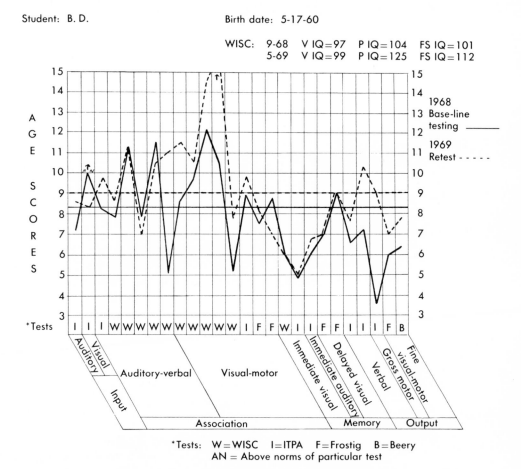

FIG. 5-6. Profile of child with type III learning disability—severe reading problems.

firm the belief that the learning disability is primary and the emotional reaction secondary.

Test and retest results are presented graphically in Fig. 5-6. It is apparent that there is no clear-cut pattern of variability in his learning profile. He is proving to be above average to superior in high-level performance skills as measured by the WISC, with a performance IQ of 125. Verbal skills measure in the average range, with verbal IQ of 99. His full-scale IQ is 112. It is interesting that circumscribed cross modality deficits continue to be present. Both auditory and visual short-term memory skills are markedly deficient. Arithmetic symbolization ability is impaired, and there continue to be some indicants of perceptual deficits, as measured by the Frostig subtests of figure-ground perception, eye-hand coordination, spatial relations, and position in space, as well as by the Beery Test of Perceptual Development. Speech and hearing testing, and complete ophthalmological testing of vision found him to be in the normal range in all these respects. By the end of his first year at Miriam School his teacher reported:

> Bob is severely limited academically by his inability to retain letter or number symbols. He is able to add with carrying and to subtract using concrete aids but does not comprehend "more'" or "less," read numbers above 10, or reproduce any numbers consistently without a model. He is able to decode three-letter words by using sound-picture clues. He does not recognize more than 5 words by sight. He is unable to recognize or reproduce the letters of the alphabet consistently without a model. He is well informed in general information relating to social studies and enters enthusiastically into class discussions. His attention and concentration are very limited, and he is easily discouraged in the classroom.

Medication continued to be of inestimable help in increasing his attention span. During the course of the year he proved to have many leadership qualities, and was liked and sought after by peers. He was physically adept and skilled at athletics.

To meet his special needs, the teacher worked with him on an individual basis in the specific areas of deficit, particularly with respect to immediate memory, both visual and auditory. One-to-one work was also carried on to develop the deficit perceptual skills measured on the Frostig test. All of this special work was done simultaneously with reteaching and beginning over again in both reading and arithmetic. In reading, the Fernald techniques of using the tactile sense through tracing and then writing (handwriting was intact for him) were initiated. A major breakthrough came with the discovery that he could, through the use of pictures, retain sounds and letters. The same picture was always used to represent the same sound—for example, the letter *b* was always represented by a picture of a baby. In this tedious, slow manner he would sound out three-letter words and then manage to build up picture memory cues that would enable him to sight-read the previously learned three-letter word without the picture present. This approach was used throughout the summer in tutoring sessions conducted four times a week. About the middle of the summer we could see some confidence building, and he was able to retain most of what he had learned. However, the progress was not steady; there were periods of regression and some loss of skills. Fortunately, for the most part the gains outweighed the losses. At no time was he required to participate in oral reading with a group, and in his one-to-one work he whispered, so that only he and the teacher could hear him. At the same time, number skills were being worked with on a very concrete basis, with the help of scored number rods and a counting frame to aid him. This too was slow and tedious work.

During his second year at Miriam School he gained enough skills for the teacher to be able to make good use of tapes through the following technique: The teacher records a story that is appropriate to the reading level of the child. The child listens with earphones to the teacher's recording, following the story word by word with a marker. The child then reads the story aloud with the teacher's tape recording, again following the words with a marker. Then he will read it over aloud and record his reading, listen back, and read it over together with his tape. At this point he may well read it aloud to the teacher, without any of the tape aids. This method helped him become free and to gain assurance that he could move along, to the point that the teacher reported the following:

> Bob is open and free in the classroom and no longer so anxiety ridden. He is not afraid of making mistakes and is now convinced that he *can* read and do academic work successfully. He is a happy child who actually seems to enjoy every minute of school and to take real pride in his work.

By the end of this second year he was achieving at a low second grade level. For the first time he was able to cope with formal achievement testing, with the following results: word knowledge, grade 2.7; word discrimination, grade 2.8; reading comprehension, grade 1.9; arithmetic, grade 3.9. At long last, he was making steady progress. Tutoring has continued during the present summer, and he will return for one more year at Miriam School, with the goals of solidifying gains and seeing whether it will be possible for him to move out of the illiterarcy class. Only time will tell how much "catching up" he will be able to do. Most boys of his present age are achieving at fourth to fifth grade level and are well on their way to being literate, to using the skill as a tool for knowledge rather than concentrating on the tool per se. Bob has come a long way, but there can be no doubt that he is a youngster with a type III learning disorder, with particular problems in reading symbols—a disorder that in our particular culture results in a major handicap for a child.

IN-SERVICE TRAINING

An important aspect of Miriam's program is concerned with ongoing in-service training of both professional staff and volunteers.

TRAINING OF PROFESSIONALS—MIRIAM STAFF. Professional staff meetings are held twice weekly after school. The regular staff is always present, with the alternate inclusion of Miriam psychiatric and educational consultants. Discussion focuses on behavioral and learning changes that occur in the children at school, at home, and in the community. Attention is given to new teaching concepts and procedures.

Experimentation with new approaches by the teachers is welcomed, and the decision to try new approaches is up to the individual teacher.

From time to time, special attention is given to some particular phase of the program and a concentrated phase of in-service training is developed. For instance, in 1964, when the decision was made to begin enrolling preschool and kindergarten children, two years of concentrated study were focussed on how best to create a program for such children. This particular study was made possible by a small grant that made available additional staff and consulting time for observation and exploration of preschool teaching techniques that might be useful for a handicapped group. The results of this in-service training were many and varied, but a primary result was a complete shift in the teaching approach, with a movement away from an open-ended preschool teaching philosophy to a definite structure, encompassing the beliefs set forth previously in this chapter. A more detailed summary of these preschool practices is given in a recent publication (Kenney, 1969). A later consequence of this in-service training was the production of a documentary film, *Thursday's Children,* to be used for purposes of community education with regular preschool and kindergarten teachers. Currently, the staff is in the process of investigating the applicability of behavioral modification techniques to Miriam School children. Again, the staff is planning to learn such techniques on a pilot basis to determine the usefulness of such a systematic charting and goal-setting approach. This pilot study will involve Miriam staff and outside specialists in the techniques of training teachers in behavioral analysis and modification.

TRAINING OF PROFESSIONALS—PRACTICE TEACHERS AND SOCIAL WORK STUDENTS. A correlate of university training programs for teachers who will work with LD and ED children in public education is well-supervised practice teaching experiences. For the past three years practice teachers from Southern Illinois University have rotated through the Miriam program, spending a quarter working with particular teachers and classrooms. This is an encouraging development, holding high hopes for meeting the needs of many more children than can enroll at Miriam School. In addition, school social workers are becoming cognizant of the importance of their role in meeting the needs of LD children. Consequently, we are currently evaluating and planning a training program that will involve working for a school year with a social work student who is in his final year of training.

TRAINING OF VOLUNTEERS. Volunteer services have proved to be an important part of the program. Full details about enlistment, training, supervision, and evaluation of volunteers are available in the 1969 Miriam School *Volunteer Handbook.*

The ongoing development of a strong corps of volunteers results in the following special benefits to the total program—benefits that cannot be secured in any other way. The children, as they prove to be ready for new experiences, have the opportunity to meet, adjust to, and understand more people. The teachers are afforded the opportunity of more effectively meeting the many individual learning and behavioral needs of the children. Knowledgeable and experienced volunteers serve as important public relations agents in the community, explaining the philosophy, methods, and learning goals of the school.

Training includes an orientation workshop, advanced workshops at various intervals, and regular supervision by the teaching staff. The purpose, for the volunteer, of the supervisory meetings held every six to twelve weeks is twofold: to discuss and understand the children's behavioral and learning progress; and to understand the particular teaching needs of each child. The purpose of such supervision for the teaching staff is to continually evaluate how well the volunteers are performing. The following questions are regularly asked about each volunteer: Is she becoming too emotionally involved with a child? Does she feel comfortable working with children? Is she enjoying her job? How do children react to her? What should be done if she is not working out? Experience has proved that most poor volunteers weed themselves out. If a situation arises in which children are not being helped or in which staff relations are being upset by a volunteer's attitude, the director deals with the problem by talking directly with the volunteer. The volunteer project's success appears to depend on maintaining an "open door" policy so that the volunteer feels free to ask for help from the director or staff. Thus the situation is met at the moment help is needed. With the utmost tact and understanding, the unsuitable volunteer must be discouraged and the eager but weak volunteer placed in a nonsensitive area.

As the needs of LD children are met in public education, there is an urgent need for training persons to work with children in regular school settings. Our fine experience with volunteers strongly suggests the benefits to be derived from such a training program. The measure of success directly relates to the care exercised in training and supervising such personnel. Any such program requires ample time from the professionals involved if maximum results are to be expected.

HOME-SCHOOL RELATIONS

All children enrolled at Miriam School live in their own homes, and parent participation in the program is important. An overall goal is for the learning and behavior patterns that develop at Miriam School to become the established patterns that are seen at home and in the community. Parental understanding is a keystone to realizing this goal. There are many avenues of communication with the home, ranging from the informal telephone or drop-in conversation with the director or the parent consultant to the regularly arranged group discussions and conference meetings.

In general, most parents become very much involved with the school and seek in every way to cooperate. Initially, many parents are anxious about participating in a special program, and some are concerned about the stigma that may be attached or skeptical of the benefits to be derived. As the child and parents become involved, anxiety and skepticism usually diminish. By the time a child is ready to leave the program, most parents begin to experience fear that gains made in learning abilities and behavior patterns will not hold in a new school setting. Consequently, the counseling needs of parents vary with the point in time and their feelings about the school. Efforts at first have to be directed toward helping them understand our goals and accepting us as partners in the joint endeavor of meeting the child's needs. At the final point, they have to be weaned from dependence on us, with full recognition by them that they are able to help the child maintain and continue to make gains—academically, socially, and emotionally.

The regular biweekly mothers' discussion groups are a major form of communication, enabling the school to know whether the child is behaving and learning at home as he is at school. Classrooms are completely visible, and parents are free to observe through one-way windows at any time. Progress and change are then the subject of discussion at the mothers' groups. At specified intervals parents meet with the director to discuss academic progress and a child's particular learning profile. Teacher-parent conferences are held twice yearly to further an understanding of learning patterns and behavioral growth.

A parent association holds four to six evening meetings a year for the purpose of keeping all parents informed of the program and offering them the chance to hear firsthand from the school consulting staff, both psychiatric and educational, and the school special therapists. The fathers have requested a couple of meetings a year with the school psychiatrist, and this avenue of communication is being explored. From the parent association arose an action group that has been instrumental in the founding of the Missouri Association for Children with Learning Disabilities. This statewide organization, now in its third year, has been in large part responsible for the passage of legislation at the state level that makes available funds for services and classrooms to meet the needs of school-age children with behavioral disorders and learning disabilities. It was this legislative action, in turn, that caused Miriam School to direct attention to the preschool and kindergarten child, and to phase out services for school-age children, who should now be served by public education.

COMMUNITY-SCHOOL RELATIONS

WHEN A CHILD IS AT MIRIAM SCHOOL. During the time a child is a student at Miriam School, close communication is maintained with community agencies and professionals involved with the child and family. About a third of the school's population is involved in some form of psychotherapy with outside family agencies, clinics, or privately practicing professionals. At regular intervals these professionals are asked to attend Miriam School staff meetings when the school psychiatrist is present. This is done with full knowledge of the child and family. Teachers at Miriam School share their knowledge about the child with the outside professionals. All professionals are welcome to observe the classrooms in action, and in many instances this firsthand knowledge has led to increased insight for the staff as well as for the visiting agencies. We have come a long way in developing interdisciplinary communication. The degree of communication that occurs seems to be directly related to the freedom to ask questions and to be able to cut through the differences in jargon of the varied disciplines. When children are receiving some form of medication, the school maintains contact with the physician in charge, sometimes directly and at other times through the parent. Careful records are kept of changes that occur in behavior, and the observations are made available to the doctor.

While the child is in attendance at Miriam School, the family is counseled to keep the child in contact with community activities, such as recreational YMCA or YWCA programs, scouts, or Indian guides. The amount and kind of involvement recommended depends on the particular behavioral or learning difficulties a child may have. Close contact with these community agencies is maintained by the school. Summer planning and programs are also included in the school's oversight of the child's total experience. Experience has proved that many Miriam School youngsters benefit greatly from being with normal and larger groups of children in well-structured summer recreation programs. For the LD children, who need special continuing remedial help in learning areas, a tutorial program at Miriam School is planned to ensure as little regression in learning skills as possible during the summer. At the same time, group camp experiences in community programs are also recommended, with tutoring hours tailored to accommodate the hours of the community recreation programs. Close contact is maintained with the recreation staff members, and their observations about the adjustment of particular youngsters serve as helpful yardsticks in determining whether growth gained at Miriam School during the school year holds and is, furthermore, transferred to a more normal setting.

Because it has not been possible to find a suitable program for some of the younger children, Miriam School has from time to time set up group recreation programs in the summer for them.

PLACEMENT AFTER LEAVING MIRIAM SCHOOL. Most children leaving Miriam School return to regular public or private schools. A number enter special public

TABLE 5-1. School placement of children after leaving Miriam School

| TYPE OF SCHOOL PLACEMENT | NUMBER OF STUDENTS | | | |
	MALE	FEMALE	TOTAL	PERCENTAGE
Regular public school	26	10	36	47
Regular private school	16	4	20	26
Special public school	5	1	6	8
Special private school	4	0	4	5
Educable mentally retarded class	4	2	6	8
Residential institution	3	0	3	4
No school	1	1	2	2
Totals	59	18	77	100

school classrooms for emotionally disturbed or learning-disordered children of normal intelligence. A few of the children admitted to the preschool prove not to have normal intellectual potential and, at the time of attaining school age, are entered into educable retarded programs in public special education. A few have been referred for residential treatment. Table 5-1 gives summary statistics about school placement of those children whose parents responded to the June, 1970, follow-up.

Most students remain at Miriam School for two years, although a few are returned to regular education at the end of a year. The decision that a child is ready to leave Miriam School is based on many factors, with major considerations related to social adjustment at school and in the community; ability to cope with learning tasks in school; and level of academic skills achieved in relation to estimated intellectual potential. When the child has been observed for a considerable period of time to be "in gear" and maintaining continued equilibrium, a judgment is then made with respect to the recommendation of optimum placement in a larger classroom. This judgment is based on facilities available within a particular school district or within the special school district. Inasmuch as in St. Louis County there are twenty-five separate school districts, all with varied sizes of classrooms and different kinds of special services, it is necessary to secure full information about a particular district at a particular time. Should some aspect of special education services appear to be appropriate, it is further necessary to investigate placement in the Special District of St. Louis County, which serves all the school districts in the county. In the event the child resides in the city of St. Louis, it is necessary to explore kinds of regular and special classrooms that are available. When a family wishes to consider private school placement, private resources are investigated.

The approach made by the Miriam staff to a given school or district will be determined by how enlightened a particular district appears to be about children who have special needs. It is apparent that more and more public school personnel are gradually becoming aware of, and are beginning to understand, the needs of LD children. Unfortunately, however, there are still some principals and teachers who have intolerant attitudes toward any child who has received specialized treatment. Experience suggests that underlying this intolerance, there is frequently a feeling of being threatened because of lack of knowledge and ability to work and plan for individual differences.

Consequently, the public relations aspects of returning a child to the normal flow of education are many, varied, and of utmost importance for the welfare of the child. The major goal, of course, is to find the best possible classroom placement for a child. To achieve this goal, many subordinate goals need to be considered, not the least of which is, in the process, to educate and inform the schools and community agencies serving the child. Such education takes the form of conferences held with school personnel and clearly written reports about the child's learning abilities, with nonjargon interpretation of the child's best way of learning and of being helped to achieve. Copies of the final report of a child are sent to the school, any agency or professional involved in therapy with the child and family, and the child's pediatrician. Experience indicates that this enhancement of communication about LD children as they resume their places in the community is a slow but meaningful way of increasing community acceptance and awareness of the particular needs of these children.

FOLLOW-UP OF ALUMNI. Each year a two-page questionnaire is sent to the parents and teachers of children who have left the school. Information is gained about social development, academic achievement, and emotional adjustment. This kind of follow-up is at best gross. The fact that not all families respond means that valuable information about a number of children is missing. Nevertheless, the trends that are suggested are of interest. It has been possible to maintain contact with 64% of the families—72 out of 112 families whose children were enrolled at Miriam School between 1962 and 1969. In addition, it was possible in June, 1970, to secure returns from 47% of the children's present teachers. Table 5-2 gives some of the comparative data secured on these questionnaire returns.

It is apparent that more youngsters are able to get along better with adults than with peers, in the estimation of both parents and teachers. However, a majority of the children are seen by both parents (67%) and teachers (64%) as functioning well with other children. In academic achievement 24% of the children do above average work in language arts and 19% do well in mathematics. There are a sizable number of children who do average work in academic subjects—45% in mathematics and 35% in language arts. Unfortunately, about a third of the population have serious academic difficulties, ranging from failure to barely passing in language arts (41%) and in mathematics (36%). It has been significant to note the increase through the years in the number of children who run into problems at higher grade levels. Comparison of present data with past data indicates that the older the child, the more likely he will be to encounter academic diffi-

TABLE 5-2. Follow-up questionnaire data of June, 1970, about students enrolled at Miriam School from September, 1962, to June, 1969

QUESTIONNAIRE ITEM	TEACHER RATINGS N = 53			PARENT RATINGS N = 72		
	1	2	3	1	2	3
Is the child happy?	76%	24%	0%	72%	22%	6%
Ability to get along						
With peers	64%	25%	11%	67%	32%	1%
With adults	81%	13%	6%	85%	14%	1%
Academic achievement levels						
Language arts	24%	35%	41%			
Mathematics	19%	45%	36%			
Emotional adjustment rating	44%	30%	26%	41%	43%	16%

culties. These difficulties seem to be of sufficient degree to suggest that there are those LD youngsters who may need special help in higher grades in school, who will prove to be unable to fit into a highly academically oriented high school curriculum. Such youngsters should have special counseling at an early point in selecting and developing skills for future vocational placement. Many of these students who prove to have serious academic problems should be able to function very well in adult years, given appropriate and timely vocational planning.

In emotional adjustment ratings, both parents and teachers perceive about a third of the children as emotionally well adjusted. Teachers see the remainder of the population as less well adjusted than do the parents. One might conjecture that the student who is not achieving academically may be perceived as less well adjusted by the teacher, whose attitude toward a student may be influenced by how well he is learning. Also, it is often difficult for a poorly achieving child to maintain a positive self-concept in the school setting, and the consequence may well be the development of secondary emotional disturbance.

A COMMUNITY EDUCATION PROGRAM FOR EARLY IDENTIFICATION OF HIGH-RISK CHILDREN

The expansion of the Miriam program to meet the needs of preschool and kindergarten-age children led to the development of a community education program with a twofold goal: early identification of high-risk children, and the education of nursery and kindergarten teachers in learning disability concepts and curriculum planning. It is hoped that through such a community education program many young children will be helped to remain in regular education and, at the same time, be taught in a manner that will allow them to compensate for learning process deficits.

A number of approaches have been used in developing this community education program, including large group meetings, informal, small discussion meetings with preschool teachers, and formal and extended workshops for varied kinds of personnel involved with young children. Participants in the workshops have included nursery school teachers and directors, a pediatrician, occupational therapists, and pediatric nurse-practitioner trainees. The concept of training nurses to help in pediatricians' offices and in clinics is an innovaton originally conceived and developed by Silver et al. Training extends over a year's time. The week spent by nurse-practitioner trainees at Miriam School was for the purpose of familiarizing them with educational concepts related to children with learning and emotional problems and making them knowledgeable in the area of atypical growth patterns. Included in the nurses' skills should be the ability to judge a child's developmental progress in a number of dimensions. The nurse could then become a major help to the pediatrician by counseling parents about atypical growth patterns and recommending referral for evaluation in depth when development is significantly skewed.

As Miriam School's community education program has grown, a network of relationships has developed between the Miriam staff and a wide range of community professionals involved in the education of young children. Consultation is frequently sought from our staff on many questions, among which are the following: When is a pattern of behavior significantly atypical? When should referral for further evaluation be made? How should parents be counseled by preschool personnel? What kind of restructuring at a school can be carried out in order to help the child compensate for particular developmental lags? It is important that preschool personnel learn the answers to these questions. Kindergartens, nursery schools, and day care centers are truly the front line of defense in that they could make possible optimum preacademic experiences, leading to the best timing for the acquisition of basic academic skills. The kind of follow-through then experienced by high-risk children as they move into regular school will be of great importance to them as well as to education in general. The passage of the Children With Specific Learning Disabilities Act of 1969 could lead to educational changes that would result in all teachers' paying more than lip service to the idea of teaching to individual differences.

Public school program development

TEACHER TRAINING PROGRAMS

It is the responsibility of institutions of higher learning to train competent personnel in special education. The federal government has played an important role in stimulating training programs for personnel working with varied kinds of handicapped children. In 1958 the passage of public law 85-926 provided for financial support for preparing personnel in the areas of mental retardation. This act was twice amended and expanded to include the training of personnel serving children with all types of handicaps. Progress in the training of personnel to work with LD children has occurred but not at a rate commensurate with need. In 1966 eleven institutions of higher education were awarded federal funds by the United States Office of Education to help support the training of personnel in the field of learning disabilities. By 1970 the Division of Training Programs of the Bureau of Education of Handicapped Children, United States Office of Education, provided funds for training in the area of learning disabilities to thirty colleges and universities. Twenty-three of the grants were for programs at the masters level or above, four were program planning grants, and three grants were for traineeships and a special summer institute.

It is significant that three years ago the Council for Exceptional Children, the professional organization concerned with the education of handicapped children, witnessed the formation of a separate Division of Children With Learning Disabilities. This division includes many disciplines but is primarily representative of teachers in special education, either classroom teachers or individual diagnostic remedial teachers.

Kass and Chalfant review the status of the training of teachers and specialists in the area of learning disabilities. They note the range of levels of training, from the introduction of the concept at the undergraduate level, to the training of remedial teachers at the masters level, to doctoral-level students who are being trained in research, college teaching, and the development and supervision of teacher training programs, as well as to assume leadership roles in various service agencies. Training programs vary from university to university but have a common core of objectives consisting of educational assessment, remedial procedures, and practicum experience.

As these training programs have developed there have been many ways in which course work and practicum experience have been related to the core objectives. A serious attempt is currently underway to clarify and exchange ideas about what optimum training of LD teachers should include. To this end an Advanced Institute for Leadership Personnel in Learning Disabilities was held at the University of Arizona in December, 1969. This institute brought together a select number of top-level professionals involved in training and service programs concerned with LD children. The final report of ideas forthcoming from this meeting was recently published by the Department of Special Education of the University of Arizona (Kass).

An important consequence of the increasing interest in training special educators to work with LD children should be a cross fertilization of LD concepts with concepts found in the field of regular education. The teacher in the regular classroom, in many instances, can be the one to solve many LD problems, given a grasp of LD theory and the courage to try new curriculum approaches with children who do not fit the mold.

DIFFERENCES AMONG PUBLIC-SCHOOL DISTRICTS

There is a wide range of differences among services available for LD children in public school districts. Much depends on the degree of recognition of LD problems that exists at a state level. If state funds become available for classes of LD children, there will follow services for such children in enlightened school districts. The degree of enlightenment, in many instances, has been directly related to the pressure of parents. The development of the parent movement in various states, under the guidance of the National Association for Children with Learning Disabilities, has played an important role in the push for legislation that has resulted in the establishment of special services and classrooms for LD children.

The special services that have resulted include diagnostic clinics relating to regular classroom teachers; diagnostic clinics relating to both regular and special classroom; resource centers in regular schools; and the work of various kinds of special remedial teachers, such as itinerant teachers who help with visual-motor skills and others that tutor in language development. Some schools have what are called developmental skills teachers—remedial teachers who work with children in relation to particular learning process deficits and basic skill difficulties. This role is often assumed by guidance counselors. Some of these special teachers work with individual children, and some work with the classroom teacher, helping her plan programs for particular children. Consequently, there is great variability at the present time in the roles and skills of special teachers.

Prior to the development of the LD concept, school districts often had speech and remedial reading teachers who would work in one or more schools. In many school systems remedial reading was never recommended until the end of third grade, by which time many nonreading youngsters had developed emotional problems. The belief that the LD child has learning process deficits has led many special educators to recommend early intervention and help in preacademic skills. It has also led to the recommendation that older children with reading problems should be tutored not only in reading but also in the development of underlying learning processes identified as deficient. This new thinking has not been absorbed by some remedial reading teachers. The combining of the knowledge and skills of the trained remedial reading teacher with LD concepts can add in important dimension to her tutoring skills. The more progressive developmental reading teachers have incorporated these challenging ideas. In the instance of speech teachers, they have in the past largely worked with speech rather than language problems, and their training has usually been in the area of speech and hearing. The LD concepts have led to the development of language specialists and have added an important dimension to speech therapy. However, many speech therapists still continue to deal only with speech problems. In some school districts, there is a whole new breed of special teachers that are developing skills in teaching language to both individuals and groups of children in regular school settings.

Further clarification of optimum services is necessary in order for school districts to be able to meet the needs of LD children. Obviously it is both unrealistic and unnecessary for public education to think only in terms of the small special classrooms that are possible on a pilot plan basis in a small private school. Insofar as possible, children should remain in regular classrooms. The process of labeling and segregating children is a serious business and should not be done without ample evidence of the need for it. A significant countermovement to the formation of special classes for many handicapped children, particularly the educable mentally retarded, was sparked by Dunn in 1968. His remarkable stand, after training special teachers of mentally retarded children for twenty years, started rumblings that may alter the face of special education for years to come. The end result of his thinking would be to do away with labeling and segregating, and to stimulate teaching to individual differences in the regular classrooms. Be that as it may, special education personnel should particularly resist the pressure to form many segregated classes for LD children and should instead push to have regular education meet the needs of most LD children with the help of varied kinds of special services. Given sufficiently early identification of problems and clarification of which children have hard-core "specific learning disabilities," it should be possible to sort out those comparative few who need to be removed to special classrooms. Appropriate learning environments should then be supplied for the many more who can be helped while being maintained in the flow of regular education.

Regular and special education are still a long way from being able to supply appropriate learning environments to meet the many different needs of children.

The key to achieving such a goal lies in developing more teachers who truly teach to individual differences and in maintaining classroom size at a level that makes it possible for a teacher to personalize teaching.

AN EVOLVING PLAN FOR CHILDREN WITH LEARNING DISABILITIES

The heterogeneity of the children who are included in the LD population is great. As special and regular education recognizes their needs, inevitably more and more children will be thought of as LD children. It is vital that we begin to make more refined distinctions among categories of disabilities and, given the distinctions, to plan in specific ways to meet the different educational needs of the children. We believe that most children's learning problems are due to poor teaching environments rather than to any inherent learning process deficit. If this is true, then it is necessary to develop some systematic way to teach to individual differences, as well as to sort out, at as early an age as possible, those youngsters who need the highly specialized help of a small classroom. Adelman has conceptualized just such a solution to meeting the needs of his proposed types I, II, and III learning disorder groups, referred to at the beginning of this chapter.

It will be recalled that type III children have major disorders in learning processes, those that could be termed "specific learning disabilities." Type II children have minor learning process disorders and, given the appropriate learning environment, can readily compensate for them. Type I students have learning problems caused entirely by poor learning environments. In Fig. 5-7 is set forth Adelman's conceptualization of sequential and hierarchical teaching strategies related to the three general categories of disorders. He hypothesizes that a personalized learning environment would be able to solve most learning problems of youngsters in the type I category. The phrase "personalized learning environment" refers to a classroom structured on a plan that allows each child to move at his own pace, and that does not set up the usual three-level group classroom, based on basal text oriented approach to teaching. It is significant that Adelman has been able to help teachers of large classrooms (thirty-five to forty children) plan personalized programs.

Built into personalized teaching is the opportunity for the teacher to employ sequential and hierarchical remedial strategies with particular children as the need arises. In the teaching process, then, the teacher is both identifying the type of learning problem that is present and planning remediation. When a child does not respond to a personalized learning environment, in which the focus has been on basic school skills and subjects, the teacher will then shift into dealing with him as a child with a type II disorder, first reteaching basic school subjects and only later, if necessary, moving into specific remediation of underlying learning processes that may be impeding formal learning. In turn, then, those youngsters who prove to have chronic disorders and who have responded to none of these remedial approaches will be the ones referred for placement in special small

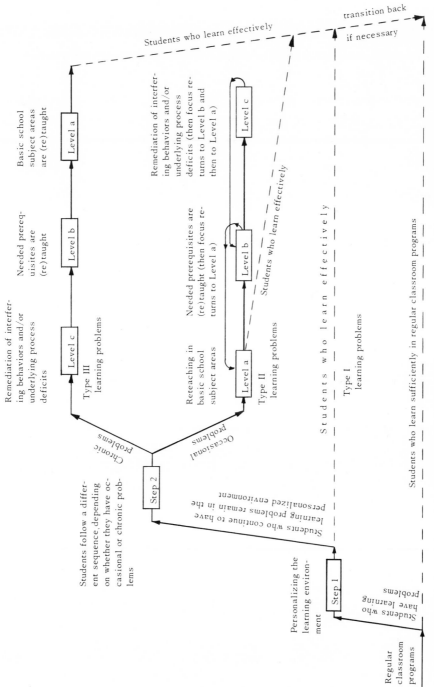

FIG. 5-7. Sequential and hierarchical teaching strategies for remedying school learning problems. (From Adelman, H. S.: The not-so-specific learning disability population, Except. Child. 37:528, March, 1971.)

classrooms. These children have type III disorders, and the remedial approach to the skill problem is reversed, with the focus on learning process remediation rather than on the basic skill itself. Those basic skills of type III students which are intact would, of course, be worked with on an instructional basis. For example, if a child has a severe reading disorder, remedial focus would be on relevant learning processes, but, if arithmetic computation skills are intact, instruction would proceed at a normal rate in this intact skill.

This sequential and hierarchical concept of teaching is of particular significance with the delay in the use of special techniques for learning process remediation until a child has clearly proved to have hard-core learning disabilities. There is a great need at the present time for research to determine what technique at what point in time can be most helpful to what kinds of children. A plethora of materials has resulted from the concept of teaching to learning process strengths and weaknesses. Some teachers, under the guise of carrying out personalized teaching, use these materials for all children in the classroom. One wonders if this is wasteful of classroom time for those students who really do not need the extra stimulation of various sensory processes. In the creation of personalized teaching structures, maximum use should be made of the talents and know-how of trained specialists in language development, visual-motor training, and developmental reading.

Both regular and special education are a long way from being able to supply personalized teaching environments of the kind conceptualized by Adelman. The key to realizing such a structure lies in developing more teachers who know what it means to teach to individual differences on the basis of the learning styles of various children. There is going to have to be a revolution in American education. The time is ripe for personnel in special and regular education to plan programs that will be sufficiently flexible from the very beginning to meet the broad spectrum of individual differences in every classroom. For instance, at the initial point of beginning to learn to read, the best method of teaching a particular child should be determined. Why should a whole class learn by either the sight method or phonics? Some children do best with one method or the other, and some need a combination of both. With this approach the teacher would not be thinking in terms of three groups on different levels of "Dick and Jane" but, instead, would be thinking in terms of varied methods that would be used with different groups and individuals. The possibility of allowing for this degree of flexibility in most regular classes is remote, but surely it should not be entirely out of the question. If a great part of the LD population—types I and II—are to be maintained in regular classrooms where they belong, such flexibility is essential.

Again, the desired flexibility should make it possible for poor readers and nonreaders to continue to learn without having to go on plugging, hour after hour, at the basic skill. Education has been revolutionized through the use of all sorts of audiovisual materials, many of which can be imaginatively adapted for individual programming. Tapes, records, language machines, movies, and filmstrips open up many avenues for making learning exciting and available to the nonliterate child. Illiteracy does not necessarily mean that the child is stupid, although in the American mind and in American education the two have usually been considered synonymous. The history of education makes it understandable why this is so. Initially, the only efficient way of learning was through the written word, and until fairly recently, this method was appropriate for most students in America who obtained a formal education. During colonial times only the socially elite or unusually gifted were formally educated—approximately 10% were afforded such an opportunity. By the end of World War II the average person had completed ninth grade, with college educations open only to a comparative few. Today, almost all children complete ten years of school, and over half the high school graduates enroll in college!

The curriculum model is going to have to broaden, because a standardized education can no longer accommodate the wide range of individual differences that will inevitably be found in such a varied population. The LD concept, educational theories, and methods will serve as an important stimulus for achieving the goal of personalized teaching that will recognize and teach to individual differences within the mainstream of regular education.

REFERENCES

Adelman, H. S.: The educationally handicapped child: some thoughts regarding who he is, why he is, and what to do about him, Keynote address, fourth annual Phi Delta Kappa Conference for the Educationally Handicapped, University of Redlands, March, 1970.

Adelman, H. S.: The not-so-specific learning disability population. In Out of the Classroom, Excep. Child. 37:528, March, 1971.

Ashlock, P., and Stephen, A.: Educational therapy in the elementary school, Springfield, Ill., 1966, Charles C Thomas, Publisher.

Ayers, J.: Tactile functions, their relation to hyperactive and perceptual-motor behavior, Amer. J. Occup. Ther. 6:6, 1964.

Barsch, R. H.: A movigenic curriculum, Madison, Wisc., 1965, Bureau for Handicapped Children.

Beery, K. E., and Buktenica, N.: Developmental Test of Visual-Motor Integration, Chicago, 1967, Follett Educational Corp.

Bessell, H., and Palomares, V.: Methods in human development, San Diego, Calif., 1970, Human Development Training Institute.

Bijou, S. W., and Baer, D. M.: Child development I, a systematic and empirical theory, New York, 1961, Appleton-Century-Crofts.

Birch, H. G.: Brain damage in children, Baltimore, 1964, The Williams & Wilkins Co.

Burgemeister, B. B.: Psychological techniques in neurological diagnosis, New York, 1962, Harper & Row, Publishers.

Burgemeister, B. B., Blum, L., and Lorge, I.: Columbia mental maturity scale, ed. 2, Yonkers, N. Y., 1959, World Book Co.

Chalfant, J. C., and Scheffelin, M.: Central processing dysfunctions in children: a review of research, NINDS monograph no. 9, Bethesda, Md., 1969, National Institutes of Health.

Cruickshank, W. M., Bentzen, F., Ratzeburg, F. H., and Tannhauser, M.: Teaching methodology for brain-injured and hyperactive children, Syracuse, 1961, Syracuse University Press.

DeHirsch, K., Jansky, J., and Langford, W. S.: Predicting reading failure, New York, 1966, Harper & Row, Publishers.

Delacato, C. H.: The diagnosis and treatment of speech and reading problems, Springfield, Ill., 1963, Charles C Thomas, Publisher.

Doll, E. A.: Preschool Attainment Record (research ed.), Circle Pines, Minn., 1966, American Guidance Service, Inc.

Dunn, L.: Peabody Picture Vocabulary Test, Circle Pines, Minn., 1959, American Guidance Service, Inc.

Dunn, L. M.: Special education for the mildly retarded—is much of it justifiable? Excep. Child. 35:5, Sept., 1968.

Fernald, G.: Remedial techniques in basic school subjects, New York, 1943, McGraw-Hill Book Co.

Fowler, W.: The effect of early stimulation. In Hess, R. D., and Bear, R. M., editors: Early education, Chicago, 1968, Aldine Publishing Co.

Friedus, E.: Methodology for the classroom teacher. In Hellmuth, J., editor: The special child in century 21, Seattle, 1964, Special Child Publications of the Seguin School.

Frostig, M.: Frostig Developmental Test of Visual Perception, Palo Alto, Calif., 1963, Consulting Psychologists Press.

Getman, G. N.: How to develop your child's intelligence, ed. 6, Luverne, Minn., 1962, G. N. Getman.

Getman, G. N., and Kane, E. R.: Developing learning readiness, St. Louis, 1968, McGraw-Hill Book Co.

Goldstein, K.: Aftereffects of brain injuries in war, New York, 1942, Grune & Stratton, Inc.

Hainesworth, P. K., and Siqueland, M.: Early identification of children with learning disabilities: the Meeting Street School screening test, Providence, 1969, Crippled Children and Adults of Rhode Island, Inc.

Johnson, D., and Myklebust, H. R.: Learning disabilities: educational principles and practice, New York, 1967, Grune & Stratton, Inc.

Kass, C.: Final report, Advanced Institute for Leadership Personnel in Learning Disabilities, Dept. of Special Education, University of Arizona, Unit on Learning Disabilities, Division of Training Programs, Bureau for the Handicapped, U. S. Office of Education, 1970.

Kass, C., and Chalfant, J. C.: Training specialists for children with learning disabilities. In Hellmuth, editor: Learning disorders, vol. III, Seattle, 1968, Special Child Publications.

Kenny, E. T.: A diagnostic preschool for atypical children. In Out of the Classroom, Excep. Child. 36:193, Nov., 1969.

Kenney, E. T.: The small classroom—a developmental idiosyncratic approach to learning and behavioral disorders in children with normal intelligence. In Inspection and introspection of special education, Council for Exceptional Children, 1964, pp. 208-217.

Kephart, N. C.: The slow learner in the classroom, Columbus, Ohio, 1960, Charles E. Merrill Publishing Co.

Kirk, S. A.: The Illinois Test of Psycholinguistic Abilities: its origin and implications. In Hellmuth, J., editor: Learning disorders, vol. III, Seattle, 1968, Special Child Publications of the Seattle Seguin School, Inc.

Kirk, S. A., McCarthy, J. J., and Kirk, W.: Illinois Test of Psycholinguistic Abilities, rev. ed., Urbana, Ill., 1968, University of Illinois Press.

Lovitt, T. C.: Assessment of children with learning disabilities, Excep. Child. 34:233, Sept., 1967.

McCarthy, J. J., and Kirk, S. A.: Illinois Test of Psycholinguistic Abilities, experimental ed., Urbana, Ill., 1961, University of Illinois Press.

McCarthy, J. J., and McCarthy, J. F.: Learning disabilities, Boston, 1969, Allyn & Bacon, Inc.

McGinnis, M.: Aphasic children: identification and education by the association method, Washington, D. C., 1963, Volta Bureau.

Mecham, J.: Verbal language development scale, Circle Pines, Minn., 1959, American Guidance Service, Inc.

Myers, P., and Hammill, D. D.: Methods for learning disorders, New York, 1969, John Wiley & Sons, Inc.

Myklebust, H. R.: Auditory disorders in children, New York, 1954, Grune & Stratton, Inc.

Orton, S. T.: Reading, writing, and speech problems in children, New York, 1937, W. W. Norton & Co., Inc.

Pick, A.: Some basic perceptual processes in reading, Young Children, **25**:162, 1970.

Redl, F.: Concept of the life space interview. In Long, N. J., Morse, W. C., and Newman, R. G., editors: Conflict in the classroom, Belmont, Calif., 1966, Wadsworth Publishing Co., Inc.

Rice, D.: Learning disabilities: an investigation in two parts, J. Learn. Dis. 3:193, April, 1970.

Roach, E. G., and Kephart, N. C.: The Purdue Perceptual-Motor Survey, Columbus, Ohio, 1966, Charles C. Merrill Publishing Co.

Silver, H. K., Ford, L. C., and Day, L. R.: The pediatric nurse-practitioner program, J.A.M.A. **204**:298-302, 1968.

Skinner, B. F.: The behavior of organisms: an experimental analysis, New York, 1938, Appleton-Century-Crofts.

Strauss, A., and Lehtinen, L.: Psychopathology and education of the brain-injured child, New York, 1947, Grune & Stratton, Inc.

Taylor, E. M.: Psychological appraisal of children with cerebral defects, Cambridge, Mass., 1961, Harvard University Press.

Terman, L. M., and Merrill, M.: Stanford-Binet Intelligence Test, Boston, 1960, Houghton Mifflin Co.

Wechsler, D.: Wechsler Intelligence Scale for Children, New York, 1949, The Psychological Corp.

Wechsler, D.: Wechsler Preschool and Primary Scale of Intelligence, New York, 1967, The Psychological Corp.

Wittes, G., and Radin, N.: The reinforcement approach, San Rafael, Calif., 1969, Dimensions Publishing Co.

chapter 6

ROLE OF THE ORTHOPTIST IN
EVALUATION OF READING DISORDERS

JANE HURTT

An orthoptist, who gives visual training to children, does not treat dyslexia but does play an important part in the preliminary steps of diagnosing this condition.

The patient is first seen by the ophthalmologist and is then referred to the orthoptist. It is the role of these two persons to determine whether or not the lack of binocular control is influencing the reading ability of the patient.

This chapter deals strictly with an orthoptic examination of all poor readers that are referred to the orthoptic clinic. For practical purposes, we have eliminated any procedures that would be carried out on preschool children.

Prior to examining the patient, the orthoptist expects a complete report from the ophthalmologist. This information should include the results of a cycloplegic refraction and a fundus examination, and the prescription of glasses, if given. It should also include the present and past history of the patient and family, and facts pertinent to the patient's present condition.

After the patient and usually a parent have entered the examining room and are seated, it is well to ask both of them a few questions so that the child can become acquainted with the examiner and will relax in the situation before the actual examination begins. Questions asked may be concerned with the age at onset of the deviation (if a deviation is present), whether the deviation is intermittent, how often the eye deviates, and the duration of the deviation each time it occurs. It is well to ask whether the condition is more noticeable to the parents as the child gets older. The patient can be questioned about whether he is symptomatic or asymptomatic. For example, does he see double, does the print blur when he reads, or do his eyes tire easily? Usually by the time the orthoptist has received this data, the patient is relaxed and cooperative.

When glasses have been prescribed, the entire examination is done while the glasses are worn, with the exception of a few tests that require the removal of the frames. (When indicated, however, the whole examination may be done without the prescription.)

THE EXAMINATION
Visual acuity

The patient is seated 20 feet from a visual acuity chart (Fig. 6-1) and is instructed to read from the top down to the smallest distinguishable letters, with each eye alternately covered. If a Project-O-Chart is used, the examiner may isolate a line of letters, starting with a large line and moving down to smaller letters,

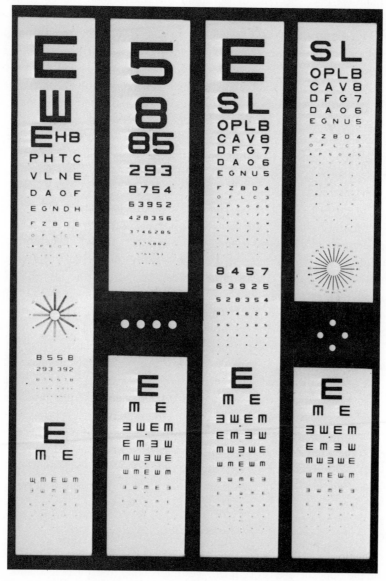

FIG. 6-1. Project-O-Chart slides. (Courtesy H. O. V. Optical Co., Inc., Chicago.)

or she may find it necessary on occasion to isolate letters to better determine the acuity of that particular patient. Acuity is recorded in fractions—for example, 20/60, 20/40, or 20/20. The smaller the denominator, the better is the acuity.

Diagnosis and measurement of deviation

There are several steps to this test, which is done at distance (20 feet) and at near (13 inches) to determine whether the deviation of the patient is a latent or manifest one, the type of deviation that exists, and the amount of deviation, measured in prism diopters.

COVER AND UNCOVER TEST. The first step is done by having the patient fixate on an object while the examiner covers one eye with an occluder and watches the uncovered eye. The covered eye is then uncovered, and the procedure is repeated several times while the examiner constantly observes the uncovered eye. This procedure is then reversed by covering and uncovering the opposite eye, always observing the uncovered eye. If the uncovered eye does not move when the opposite eye is covered (and the other eye does not move when the procedure is reversed), then the deviation is considered to be a phoria, or latent, one. If the uncovered eye does move to pick up fixation when the opposite eye is covered, the deviation is manifest.

ALTERNATE COVER TEST. The second step is to alternate the occlusion, that is, to cover the right eye and then the left eye alternately by slipping the occluder over the patient's nose from one eye to the other. During this step the examiner is constantly observing the eye that is immediately uncovered—to determine whether the eye moves out or moves in to pick up fixation. If the immediately uncovered eye moves outward, the eye was turned in under the cover, and the deviation is an esophoria or esotropia. If the eye moves inward, the eye was turned out under the cover, and the deviation is an exophoria or exotropia.

PRISM AND COVER TEST. Whether the deviation is latent (phoria) or manifest (tropia), and whether it is of the inward type or the outward type, the movement of the eyes is measured with prisms and with the alternate cover test using the necessary amount of prisms to neutralize the deviation. When this is accomplished, the amount of deviation is recorded in prism diopters.

During these three steps the examiner may also observe a vertical deviation as well as a horizontal one. This vertical deviation could be a hyperphoria, a hypertropia, a hypophoria, or a hypotropia (see Glossary at the end of chapter). The direction and amount of deviation are detected and measured in the same manner as the horizontal one.

Ductions

Ductions are the movements of one eye in all directions of gaze (see Glossary) while the opposite eye is occluded. Testing is done to determine whether full motility of all the extraocular muscles is present in all these directions.

Versions

Versions are the parallel movements of both eyes in all the cardinal directions of gaze. They are tested in connection with an alternate cover test while the patient is looking in these various directions. The test is done to detect a paresis of any of the vertical-acting muscles.

A *and* V *measurements*

This phase of the examination is done by having the patient fixate on an accommodative target at a distance of 20 feet. He is first instructed to elevate his chin so that he is looking down at the target while the examiner measures the amount of deviation. He is then asked to depress his chin so that he is now looking up at the target, and the orthoptist again measures the amount of deviation.

An esotropia with an A syndrome has a greater amount of deviation (turning in) of the visual axes looking up than looking down. An A exotropia has a greater amount of deviation (turning out) of the visual axes looking down than looking up.

A V esotropia has a greater amount of turning in when looking down, and a V exotropia exhibits a greater amount of turning out when looking up.

During this part of the examination it may be evident that a vertical deviation becomes greater in either the upward or the downward gaze. When the examiner finds a hypertropia on this test, she should also take the measurements of the upward and the downward gaze at 13 inches.

Worth 4-dot test

The worth 4-dot test is a binocular test done at distance and at near to determine whether the patient has fusion, diplopia, or suppression. The distant apparatus (Fig. 6-2) contains four holes and a lighting system. The upper hole is covered with red, the side ones are covered with green, and the lower one is covered with white. A pair of red-green glasses, the colors complementary to those on the lighted box, are worn by the patient, with the red lens in front of the right eye and the green in front of the left eye. The patient's responses may be as follows:

1. "I see two dots that are red." Indications are that the left eye is suppressed, since that is the eye covered by the green lens.

2. "There are three green dots." This indicates suppression of the right eye.

3. "Five dots. Three are green and two are red." If the two red dots are seen on the right and the three green on the left, the diplopia is homonymous (uncrossed). If the patient describes the red dots as being on the left and the green on the right, the diplopia is heteronymous (crossed).

4. "There are four dots. The top one is red, the side ones are green, and the bottom one appears mixed red and green." With this response, the patient is describing fusion and is seeing the top red dot with the right eye, the side green ones with the left eye, and the white bottom one with both eyes, mentally blended red-green.

A smaller type of this model may be used for near testing, as shown in Fig. 6-3.

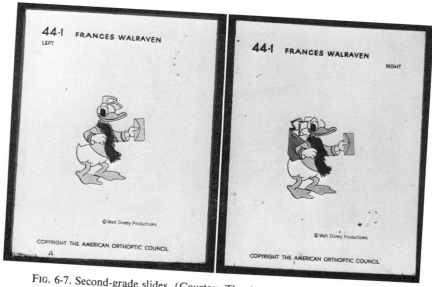

FIG. 6-7. Second-grade slides. (Courtesy The American Orthoptic Council.)

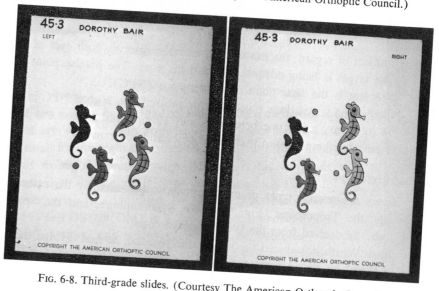

FIG. 6-8. Third-grade slides. (Courtesy The American Orthoptic Council.)

prism diopters of amplitudes. If he cannot do so, then he has only superimposed second-grade targets and has no fusion. If one of the check marks (mailbag or cap) is missing, then suppression, which may be monocular or alternating, is present. He may also, at this point, have diplopia, which may indicate either that his angle of deviation is variable or that he has no fusion ability.

THIRD-GRADE (STEREOSCOPIC VISION). The slides used in testing for this grade of fusion are identical but have a certain amount of horizontal disparity. The greater the disparity, the greater is the depth perception experienced by a patient who possesses first- and second-grade fusion. If you were able to lay one slide on top of the other in Fig. 6-8, you would notice that the sea horses would not be exactly superimposed on each other (which is the case with the Donald Duck slides); instead all the sea horses on one of the slides would be off center in relation to the other slide. However, if you were to view these slides in the major amblyoscope, one set would not appear off center. Four sea horses could be seen, one of them would appear to be a great deal closer, and the others, in order, would seem farther away in graded steps.

SIGNIFICANCE OF FINDINGS

A patient with a *constant manifest deviation* with deep suppression would not have a reading problem because of the muscle imbalance. He would be using only one eye while the other one would be suppressed. We can therefore eliminate this type from the poor reader group because he would be asymptomatic.

A *divergence excess* will result in difficulty in using the two eyes together while fixating at distance but not while reading.

Divergence insufficiency is also a condition that affects the binocular use of the two eyes at distance but not at near.

Although a *convergence excess* indicates that the patient has a greater amount of deviation at near, it does *not* mean that he will be symptomatic in the reading position. The deviation could be a manifest tropia in that position (with suppression in the deviated eye), which would not create any difficulty for him. However, he definitely would have problems in the reading position if his deviation were of the intermittent type. The patient with this condition may be reading while his eyes are straight (esophoria), and suddenly one eye may deviate inward (esotropia). In the absence of suppression of that eye, he would see double. Although he cannot explain what has happened, he has lost his place because the images of the two pages, which he has been mentally fusing, have drifted apart, and the situation has created diplopia for him. The deviation may be an esophoria and also may be stable, which would present no problems. There are other patients in this classification who may also have a latent inward deviation but *not* a reserve amount of amplitudes. This type of difficulty may produce symptoms that are described as a burning of the eyes, a blurring of the print, and severe headaches.

Probably the most common motility problem, and the one that produces the most symptoms, is the *convergence insufficiency* type. When Duane classified the types of deviations, he stressed that the exo deviation was the type that fell into the category of convergence insufficiency. It is a known fact by all in the motility field, however, that some eso deviations can also produce many symptoms because of insufficient convergence ability. It is therefore possible for a poor reader to fall into this category easily. The persons with an exo deviation, however, are usually bothered the most by reading difficulty. If they have little or no suppression, they find that doing close work for any period of time is almost impossible. On the other hand, if the patient has a great deal of suppression, he may be symptomatic only occasionally and not even be aware of his problem.

children between 2½ and 6 years of age. The subjects were required to find a picture appropriate to the initial sound. Only 50% of the 6-year-old children succeeded in the task. The ability to rhyme words was demonstrated to be quite difficult for children below 5½ years of age.

Speech as a series of acoustic stimuli

Fant reports that divergent opinions have been expressed on the nature of speech. The concept of speech as a sequence of discrete units with distinct boundaries joined together like beads on a string is contrasted to the view of speech as a continuous succession of gradually varying and overlapping patterns. In considerable detail nine parameters of speech have been designated by Fant to account for the acoustical basis of identifying sound features. The major features of speech—frequency, intensity, and rate—will be discussed. Together they comprise the major acoustical load in the perception of speech. These parameters are often controllable by the clinician.

FREQUENCY. The number of vibrations per second produced by a sound source is referred to as frequency; one cycle per second is designated as a hertz (Hz.). Human hearing encompasses a total range of approximately 20 to 20,000 c.p.s. The concern here is with the range of sound waves produced by the vocal structures, which is roughly between *125* and *8,000* Hz. (Judson et al.). Pitch is the subjective or auditory awareness of frequency. On a pitch scale, sounds can be ranked from low to high or from bass to treble. The range of human hearing is most sensitive for the frequency range of speech; the components within this frequency range, however, are not equally perceptive. Consonants are usually characterized by higher frequencies than vowels and are critical for recognition or identification of spoken words. Some sounds, such as the weak fricatives "th," "f," and "v," and the sibilants such as "s" and "z," are characterized by a high-frequency spectrum. The research of French and Steinberg indicates that the low frequencies contribute little to intelligibility even though they carry most of the speech power. Differentiation between similar high- frequency sounds—for example, the "th" and "f" sounds—may be difficult, and differences may be easily masked by background noises. The sounds "v" and "f," and the aspirated "th," account for more than half the phonetic mistakes made in the perception of normal conversation (Fletcher). The short "e," as in bed, and "i," as in hit, frequently troublesome in teaching reading, are relatively similar in frequency.

INTENSITY. The amount of energy used to produce a sound wave is referred to as intensity. The subjective, or auditory, aspect of intensity is loudness, which may be rated on a scale from soft to loud. According to Fletcher, a round figure of about 0.01 microwatt probably represents the faintest sound, and an intensity of 5,000 microwatts represents the peak value of loudest sound in conversation—a range in intensity of 500,000 to 1. The consonant sounds are characteristically weak in intensity relative to vowel sounds (Fletcher). A vowel sound in an accented syllable has usually three or four times as much phonetic power as one in an unaccented syl-

AUDITORY-ARTICULATOR

deficiencies who are les
many of the oral-facia
training focuses on th
tongue movements can
speech sound positions
musculature. Sounds t
rate, as well as those
learned with model d
facial clues can facili
lips, and soft palate a
similar sounds. Oral-f
the relation between
musculature (Fig. 7-2)

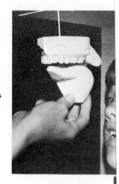

A

C

FIG. 7-2. Using a model, a
pronounced "gul." The "u"
toward the floor of the m
demonstrates the sequences
associated sounds in teachi
tongue as it makes contac
simultaneous and rapid ele
tongue is in contact with th
for the "l," the final aspec
peated at increasingly rapid

AUDITORY-AR

aurally and
articulatory
consonant,
the individ
breath plo
tively, and

In add
have diffic
the final a:
phonation
sary to eff
release of
by a very s

PARTIAL P

Difficu
in the not
an initial
may prod
into an "s
sition of t
errors nee
stages of
serve to
enabling
able to sh

Most
out speci
produced
"u," as i
when th
say "bu-
problem
before th
transitio

INTERW

At
phrasing
of ineffi
tions en
within s
in the w

AUD

de
ur
fe
ve
In
tif
an

Develo

ag
m:
6:
to
of
tal
du
ch
int

—
*F
m

lable. The most powerful sound is "o" (áwl) and the faintest, "th" (thin). In the average room in the city, when a speaker is about 10 feet from the listener, the aspirated "th" sound is barely audible (Fletcher).

RATE. The normal ear has a phenomenal capacity to perceive complex acoustical changes of speech stimuli within tenths and even hundredths of a second. During conversational speech the auditory and articulatory changes are so fast that it is usually impossible as well as unnecessary to consciously define the specific pitch and loudness events managed by the perceptual mechanisms. The ability to resolve rapidly changing acoustical stimuli into distinctive units of variable size and complexity, however, is essential for identification and recall of speech sounds for learning printed word recognition. According to Potter et al., speech sound production is so rapid that it is frequently difficult for an untrained person to recognize the individual vowels that are combined in common diphthongs. Crandall has measured the general rate of change in vowel production. There is first a period of rapid growth in amplitude that lasts about 0.04 second. During this initial rise all the components of the sound are quickly produced and rise nearly to maximum amplitude. The second, or middle, period lasts about 0.165 second, and the final period lasts about 0.09 second. The total average time for the event approximates 0.295 second. Short vowels are truly short in duration, which, in addition to similarities in frequency, accounts for difficulty in perception. The duration of the short "i," as in "hit," and the duration of the short "e," as in "bed," are approximately 0.211 and 0.219 second, respectively. The duration of the stop consonants "b" as in "ba" ranges from 0.12 to 0.19 second, and of "p" as in "pa," from 0.02 to 0.04 second. The transitional sound "dtha" varies from 0.18 to 0.20 (Fletcher). The more rapidly speech sounds are produced, the less likely is the ear able to perceive clues that characterize particular sounds. Differentiation between sounds, such as "sh" and "ch" in the words "shoe" and "chew" or "wish" and "which," is made more difficult as the rate is increased. According to Hirsh, the sound spectra for isolated "b" and "w" are very similar. If these sounds are set before the vowel "a," whether the listener hears "ba" or "wa" is determined almost entirely by the rate at which the speaker changes from one acoustic pattern to the other. The problem of identification of the letters "p," "b," "d," and "q" with sounds has been traditionally considered as visual in nature. Similarities in form and disturbances in spatial relationship or orientation have been among the common explanations of the problem. Without instrumentation careful listening to the production of the sounds as they are spoken can reveal the acoustical similarities between them: "puh" (breath), "bu" (voice), "du" (voice), and "kwh" (breath), respectively.

Potter et al. developed a system of "visible speech" by which the acoustical characteristics of sound, syllables, and words can be projected into spectrograms for analysis. Spectrograms can illustrate the similar structural basis of many of the complex sounds and transitions that sound alike. They can provide the educator with remarkable insight into the changing patterns of speech. The use of spectrograms affords an opportunity to contrast the physical nature of sounds in isola-

the
cli
fo1
un
fir
av
st:
sli
A
"i
"i
a1
cl
i1
s1
c
a
e

/

:
1
]
]
(

of words with
choppy, and
development (
in the child's
ferent speech
experience th

PERSEVERATI\

The study
sound placem
possible by an
The children,
to read unde1
the discrimina
in reading. Tl
in the area of
open bites rev
to shift place1
placement and
attack were ob
Frequently af
placement co1
final letter in
suggested a p
the initial pla
from the final
the attack of
reversals occu
monitoring co
to assume a d
sounds, and t
dramatic result

Oral-facial clues

In many (
clues, as well
between the st
deficiencies of

_____

*During the earl
—"a-e," as in "m
prescan the word
sence of the seco
respectively.

PERSPECTIVE

Monroe was one of the early pioneers to relate speech problems to deficiencies in reading. Artley reported that there appears to be a relation between speech difficulties and deficiencies in reading, although he noted a lack of agreement as to the extent of the relation. Sommers et al. found in their study that "speech therapy" did not affect reading factor scores in any significant way. We have seen that in order to start to understand the relation between speech problems and reading problems, and between auditory problems and reading problems, it is necessary first to understand the relation between auditory and articulatory functions within a specific framework of speech for reading. As a result of the close interdependence of the auditory-articulatory functions, it is often difficult to assess independently the specific operations of the auditory system and of the articulatory system. It is difficult and sometimes impractical to attempt isolation of the perceptual component in perceptual-motor function. The types of interaction between the auditory and articulatory systems change as advances are made in the hierarchy of levels in the teaching of specific reading skills. Many of the examples of disturbances reported here suggest the need for relating relatively specific problems of auditory-articulatory functioning, in toto, to relatively specific types of problems or errors in learning to read. The auditory and articulatory functions in reading are so closely dependent on each other that remediation for the underachiever or for the child with defined deficiencies, whether scattered or specific, is concerned with specialized training in speech perception within the framework of reading and is closely integrated with specialized training in the control of the oral musculature.

Children who demonstrate auditory-articulatory problems in learning printed word recognition may respond in one or more of the following ways:

1. Produce words correctly but only with struggling and delay
2. Produce similar or microdistorted words with a somewhat similar articulatory pattern of movement and acoustical pattern
3. Produce a different word
4. Produce sounds that do not form words
5. Reverse words
6. Fail to blend sounds from letters
7. Fail to learn, recognize, or recall sounds
8. Refuse to decode the word or withdraw from the task because of anticipated failure

It is possible that such tests as Wepman's Auditory Discrimination Test and the "auditory attention span for unrelated words" subtest (Baker and Leland: Detroit Tests of Learning Aptitude) may provide evidence of an auditory problem. Studies have demonstrated a positive relation between performance on Wepman's Auditory Discrimination Test and success in reading (Goetzinger et al.; Thompson). The most valuable information is limited, however, to the specific tasks evaluated by such tests. Poor performance may suggest the possibility of disturbances "related" to auditory or auditory-articulatory tasks involved in the learning of reading skills. Such tests, and others similar to them, may deal with such aspects as whole-word units, judgment, psycholinguistic functions, and longer-term memory. Poor performance on such measurements, which do not assess the specific auditory-articulatory functions for the learning of reading skills, can suggest at best only indirect and often vague recommendations for specific educational needs.

The "auditory closure" and "sound blending" subtests of the Illinois Test of Psycholinguistic Abilities were designed for assessing psycholinguistic aspects of communication (Kirk et al.). These subtests, interestingly, resemble the operations used in learning to read and may have some value in assessment of auditory-articulatory functions. Under the usual conditions of teaching, the operations of closure and blending, however, are performed with or derived from printed letters; printed letters are not presented to the subject in these tests of closure and blending. Auditory closure and blending that may involve closure are relatively intermediate functions in the hierarchy of steps in the teaching of reading. Facility for closure is helpful particularly under conditions of blending when the child fails to recall certain sounds, or if certain sounds are distorted. Children's performances on these measures appear to differ markedly, depending on the extent to which a child orally repeats word parts or sounds spoken by the examiner and his previous experience in matching sounds with letters and recalling sounds from letters. Measurements of closure and blending can have practical value in making assessments and recommendations for special training—but only after assessment and remediation, when necessary, at the more basic levels of auditory-articulatory functioning. Substantial advancements have been made in past years in using speech stimuli to make specific diagnoses of adults with auditory-perceptual problems. A brief description of these types of diagnostic tests is provided by Becker. According to Frisina, with the possible exception of the competing-message techniques used with adults, suitable tests for children have not been proposed.

The following summary of the hierarchy of auditory-articulatory functions in the learning of reading skills may serve, at least in part, as a guide for descriptive assessment and possible future development of formal evaluation procedures.

1. *Fractionated auditory-articulatory functions.* In contrast to conversation, the fractionation of words into parts necessitates changes in the auditory-articulatory processes. A unique reciprocal and dynamic relation is required between discrete positions and movements of the oral musculature, and the auditory sounds produced from them. Children vary in their ability to teach themselves fractionation and the assignment of auditory-articulatory functions to letters.

2. *Interperceptual associations.* Sounds and articulatory movements become associated with printed letters, and the letters serve as stimuli for the recalling of auditory-articulatory functions. In some situations letters are to be recalled from speech stimuli.

3. *Auditory perception of speech and articulation for isolated and blended*

complex sounds. Auditory-articulatory functions for isolated and blended complex sounds require accurate perception of rapidly changing speech stimuli of oneself and others, and rapid and accurate integration, projection, and production of the gross and fine articulatory movements.

4. *Absolute interperceptual recall.* Recall of individual sounds from printed letters is relatively free of meaningful associations and is considered to be a relatively difficult, specialized, and isolated function.

5. *Conversational operations of auditory-articulatory functions.* As the units of reading increase in size from whole words to phrases or groups of words, the auditory-articulatory functions become more similar to those in conversation.

6. *Maintenance and suppression of word attack skills.* To increase reading speed it is necessary to suppress the influences of cumbersome and time-consuming word attack operations while maintaining these skills in order to decode the continuous influx of new reading vocabulary.

Little or no attention has been given to the linguistic, psycholinguistic, or intellectual aspects that comprise an obviously essential and significant aspect in learning to read. During the early years of life the establishment and growth of language for communication is greatly dependent on auditory-articulatory development. At school age the child's language for communication serves to steer and focus auditory-articulatory development for reading. Disturbances in auditory-articulatory perceptual functions can result in deficiencies in the development of language. In circular fashion deficiencies in language, in turn, create additional burdens in learning to read. Reading and verbal communication are our two major media for attaining continuous, lifelong language growth. Auditory-articulatory functions are therefore essential to the development of language for both verbal communication and reading and, more specifically in the interest of the reading clinician, for verbal communication to learn reading. Verbal communication and reading are the two highways toward the fulfillment of the child's intelligence, and this fulfillment is the mutually shared goal of all professionals in all areas of education.

REFERENCES

Artley, A. S.: A study of certain factors presumed to be associated with reading and speech difficulties, J. Speech & Hearing Dis. 13:351, 1948.

Baker, H. J., and Leland, B.: Detroit Tests of Learning Aptitude, Indianapolis, 1967, The Bobbs-Merrill Co., Inc.

Becker, L. V.: Comments on the possibility of using modified printed linguistic stimuli in study of visual perception and its disorders, Perceptual & Motor Skills 25:81, 1967.

Birch, J., and Mathews, J.: The hearing of mental defectives, Amer. J. Men. Deficiency, **55:** 384, 1951.

Bishop, C. H.: Transfer effects of word and letter training, J. Verbal Learn. & Verbal Behavior 3:215, 1964.

Bocca, E., and Calearo, C.: Central hearing processes. In Jerger, J., editor: Modern developments in audiology, New York, 1963, Academic Press, Inc.

Bosma, J. F., editor: Symposium on oral sensation and perception, Springfield, Ill., 1967, Charles C Thomas, Publisher.

Carhart, R.: In Davis, H.: Hearing and deafness, New York, 1947, Murray Hill Books, Inc.

Crandall, I. B.: Bell System Technical Journal, Oct., 1925.

Fant, C. G. M.: Descriptive analysis of the acoustic aspects of speech, Logos 5:3, 1962.

Fletcher, H.: Speech and hearing, New York, 1929, D. Van Nostrand Co., Inc.

French, N. R., and Steinberg, J. C.: Factors governing intelligibility of speech sounds, J. Acoustical Soc. Amer. 19:1947.

Frisina, R. D.: Measurement of hearing in children. In Jerger, J., editor: Modern developments in audiology, New York, 1963, Academic Press, Inc.

Gibson, E. J., Pick, A., Ossen, H., and Hammond, M.: The role of grapheme-phoneme correspondence in the perception of words, Amer. J. Psychol. 75:554, 1962.

Goetzinger, C. P., Dirks, D. D., and Baer, C. J.: Auditory discrimination and visual perception in good and poor readers, Ann. Otol. Rhin. Laryng. 69:121, 1960.

Gray, G. W., and Wise, C. M.: The bases of speech, New York, 1946, Harper & Brothers.

Hardy, W. G.: Problems of audition, perception, and understanding, Volta Rev. 58:289, 1956.

Harrington, D. A.: Language and perception, Volta Rev. 67:191, 1965.

Hirsh, I. J.: Information processing in input channels for speech and language: the significance of serial order of stimuli. In Clark, H., and Darley, F. L.: Brain mechanisms underlying speech and language, New York, 1967, Grune & Stratton, Inc.

Judson, L. S. V., and Weaver, A. T.: Voice science, New York, 1965, Appleton-Century-Crofts.

Kirk, S. A., McCarthy, J. J., and Kirk, W. D.: Illinois Test of Psycholinguistic Abilities, Chicago, 1968, University of Illinois.

Lehiste, I., editor: Readings in acoustic phonetics, Cambridge, Mass., 1967, The M.I.T. Press.

Licklider, J. C. R., and Miller, A.: The perception of speech. In Stevens, S. S., editor: Hankbook of experimental psychology, New York, 1951, John Wiley & Sons, Inc.

Lieberman, P.: Intonation, perception, and language, Research monograph no. 38, Cambridge, Mass., 1967, The M.I.T. Press.

Milisen, R.: Methods of evaluation and diagnosis of speech disorders. In Travis, L. E., editor: Handbook of speech pathology, New York, 1957, Appleton-Century-Crofts.

Monroe, M.: Children who cannot read, Chicago, 1932, The University of Chicago Press.

Peterson, G. E., and Lehiste, I.: Duration of syllable nuclei in English, J. Acoustical Soc. Amer. 32:693, 1960.

Potter, R. L., Kopp, G. A., and Green, H. C.: Visible speech, New York, 1947, D. Van Nostrand Co., Inc.

Sommers, R. K., Cockerville, C. E., Paul, C. D., Bowser, D. C., Fichter, G. R., Fenton, A. K., and Copetas, F. G.: Effects of speech therapy and speech improvement upon articulation and reading, J. Speech Hearing Dis. 26:27, 1961.

Spencer, E.: Thesis, Evanston, Ill., 1958, Northwestern University.

Stevens, S. S., and Davis, H.: Hearing: its psychology and physiology, New York, 1938, John Wiley & Sons, Inc.

Strauss, A., and Kephart, N.: Psychopathology and education of the brain-injured child, New York, 1955, Grune & Stratton, Inc.

Templin, M. C.: Certain language skills in children, Institute of Child Welfare monograph no. 26, Minneapolis, 1957, University of Minnesota Press.

Templin, M. C., and Darley, F. L.: The Templin-Darley tests of articulation, Iowa City, 1960, Bureau of Educational Research and Service, Extension Division, State University of Iowa.

Thompson, B. B.: A longitudinal study of auditory discrimination, J. Ed. Res. 56:376, 1963.

Wellman, B. L., Case, I. M., Mengert, I. G., and Bradbury, D. E.: Speech sounds of young children, University of Iowa Studies of Child Welfare, 5, No. 2, 1931.

Wepman, J. M.: Auditory discrimination, speech, and reading, El. Sch. J. p. 325, 1960.

chapter 8

ROLE OF THE NEUROLOGIST IN MANAGEMENT OF CHILDREN WITH LEARNING DISABILITIES

HARVEY EDWARD CANTOR

More and more children are being referred to neurologists for evaluation of learning problems. Referrals come not only from pediatricians but from physical education teachers, classroom teachers, and parents. Often the note accompanying the child merely says "? organic" or "needs EEG"; however, the unexpressed hope is that the neurologist will, through some jealously treasured knowledge or technique, be able to "cure" the child of his problem. Unfortunately, no such knowledge or technique exists; however, the concerned neurologist can help significantly in the management of children with learning disabilities.

Children with learning disabilities have been said to be suffering from dyslexia, developmental dyslexia, specific learning disability, central handicap, hypokinetic syndrome, hyperactivity, minimal brain damage, minimal cerebral dysfunction, etc. The variety of descriptive terms and definitions, the implied importance of "soft" neurological signs, the claims of therapeutic success with different approaches, and the poorly designed studies in the literature have all created a great deal of confusion regarding children with learning disabilities. This confusion has led many physicians to feel inadequate to deal with these children and to conclude, erroneously, that all of them should be evaluated by a neurologist. This chapter will attempt to define learning disability, comment on its incidence and cause, and describe the behavioral characteristics common to the many children with this problem. A role for the neurologist or other physician in the management of children with learning problems will be suggested and related to the traditional medical approach of history, physical examination, laboratory studies, consultation, and treatment. Finally, areas requiring further attention and research will be mentioned.

DEFINITION OF LEARNING DISABILITY

The terms "learning disability" and "learning problems" are used interchangeably in this chapter to refer to the inability of a child with presumably normal intelligence, vision, hearing, and neuromuscular function to learn in a classroom setting at the same rate as the average student. The definition is purposely broad so as to include the majority of children referred to neurologists for evaluation of school problems. Children lacking motivation to learn and having emotional problems are not excluded, as these factors figure prominently in most learning problems and must be dealt with in successful management.

It is variously estimated that between 5% and 20% of children in elementary schools have learning disabilities. Even at a prevalence of only 5%, this problem is more frequent than the combined incidence of mental retardation (3%), cerebral palsy (0.5%), and epilepsy (0.5%). The variance in reported incidence results from lack of agreement as to definitions of learning disabilities, differences in the characteristics of the population studied, and lack of any large, well-designed population studies. Boys with learning problems outnumber girls three or four to one. The preponderance of boys with learning disabilities is a result of their somewhat slower maturation than girls and of their central nervous system being slightly more vulnerable to insult than the female central nervous system. The recent increase in referrals of children with learning problems to neurologists and other physicians is related to the great importance education has in our society, to the attention children with learning problems have attracted in our popular press, and to the desire of informed parents to seek answers to their children's problems, rather than to any real increase in the incidence of school problems.

CAUSES OF LEARNING DISABILITIES

The causes of learning problems are diverse, rarely unifactorial, and usually interrelated. Some children mature significantly later than their peers. When they are presented with the learning situation, they are unable to cope with it, and then they may become hyperactive and "aggressive," reactions that further interfere with their learning. Slow maturation may be a consequence of individual variance or may be genetically determined. The fact that some children mature socially more rapidly than others is well accepted. Thus it is somewhat surprising that the concept of large individual differences in ability or capacity to learn, perhaps secondary to variance in the rate of myelination of the central nervous system, is not widely recognized. Studies documenting differences in completeness of myelination of the central nervous system in children of the same age give an anatomical basis for differences in learning abilities observed. This point deserves stressing because it may explain the confusing claims of success reported in the literature for one approach or another in children with learning problems. A good deal of the "success" may be accounted for on the basis of further central nervous system myelination and resulting increased ability to learn, rather than on the basis of a particular device or approach. Some authorities believe that most learning problems are secondary to inherited differences in the rate of central nervous system maturation and that if the resulting differences in ability of the "slow" children are recognized early, and if the demands made on them and the techniques used in teaching them are modified, then the more recalcitrant psychological problems secondary to learning disabilities can be avoided. Other children's learning problems are undoubtedly manifestations of damage to their central nervous system occurring during pregnancy or delivery, or postnatally. These children are examples of a continuum of damage to the central nervous system that starts with perinatal deaths, continues through mental retardation and cerebral palsy to convulsive disorders and learning disabilities, and ends with normalcy. Children with low intelligence make up another sizable portion of children with learning problems. The concept of low intelligence needs redefining in relation to the situation that the child faces. A child with a "normal" IQ of 90 in a suburban school is at a distinct disadvantage academically, as his classmates' mean IQ may well be 115 or 120. Less commonly, a child with a high IQ may do poorly in school and behave in a hyperactive manner because he is bored with school and vents his frustrations by attracting attention to himself.

Another frequent cause of poor school behavior and performance is poor motivation to learn, the reasons for which are rarely obvious, require careful questioning to elicit, and may become apparent only after a relationship has been established between parents and physician. Although a father may state at the first interview that he is concerned about his son's failure in school, it may later become apparent that he had similar difficulties in school and views his son's misbehavior as "manly." The son, sensitive to his father's unexpressed feelings, is unconcerned about school. Other children learn to "use" their inability to attract the attention of their parents and teachers for the purpose of satisfying various psychological needs and are therefore motivated to "nonlearn." Exempted from most discussions regarding the causes of learning disabilities in children is the largest group of all—children from a low socioeconomic environment. Parents of such children are often unconcerned about the child's school progress. Even if the parents are concerned, the adult models available for the children to emulate are people without education. These children are often fed inadequate diets, may be exposed to toxins such as lead, and are crowded into inadequate classrooms where teachers expect little from them. All these factors contribute to the large discrepancy in achievement between children in low socioeconomic families and children in middle-class families.

BEHAVIOR CHARACTERISTICS

Children with learning disabilities have many similar behavior characteristics. These children frequently have serious behavior problems, which may be the true reason that the parents seek medical advice. Seemingly unlimited energy, continually "getting into everything," unaffectionate behavior, purposeful annoyance of siblings, inability to follow even simple requests, inattention to household rules, disorganized behavior, prolonged and rowdy temper tantrums, and instability of mood are all common complaints. These behavior characteristics are often present from early in life and cause parental rejection, anger, and resentment toward the child. When these parental emotions are added to the frustrations and disappointments that accompany a child's inability to learn in school, the child may come to view himself as stupid, different, or bad. Such views are often expressed by his parents and teachers in the height of emotional disappointment or anger, further reinforcing the child's negative self-image. At school, children with learning problems are often inappropriately or overly active and unable to attend to one task for a reasonable period of time. Extraneous noises, objects, and thoughts command their attention, interfering with their ability to concentrate and learn. They manifest their inability to concentrate by daydreaming, shifting around in their chairs, getting up and walking about the room, or acting in similar ways that are disturbing to their classmates and teachers. Often these children seem able to learn one skill, such as arithmetic, normally but fail miserably in others, especially reading and spelling. The disturbance they cause in class and their recalcitrance in learning despite seemingly normal intelligence quite naturally upsets the teacher, further complicating their problems. These children are described as awkward and clumsy and as having poor handwriting. One wonders if these problems are fairly equally distributed among all elementary-school children regardless of learning ability but are commented on only when a child has learning problems because he is scrutinized more carefully. Regardless, difficulties in handwriting only compound problems of adjustment to school. Inability to compete successfully in sports because of clumsiness lowers the child's self-expectations and heightens his discomfort in school because it is yet another area of embarrassment and failure.

MEDICAL EVALUATION

Traditionally, medical problems are approached by obtaining a medical history, performing a physical examination, ordering indicated laboratory tests, and arranging necessary consultation. The desire is that this orderly process will produce a diagnosis that indicates cause so that specific treatment can be instituted. This approach is successful with a large number of illnesses, as illustrated by the successful treatment of bacterial infections with specific antibiotics. If the goal of the neurologist in handling children with learning disabilities is merely to rule out the existence of remediable medical problems and to treat hyperactivity pharmacologically, a fairly straightforward neurological evaluation is all that is required. Unfortunately, this limited approach is rarely of benefit to the child, as effective methods of changing behavior are much more complicated. Anyone treating patients with "psychosomatic illnesses" can attest to the considerable amount of time and effort that must be devoted to the patient to help him with his problem. The more complicated the problem, the more difficult is the therapy and the greater is the investment of time required by physician and patient alike. Learning is a complex behavior and depends on intelligence, motivation, memory, intact perceptual abilities, and functioning integrative mechanisms of the central nervous system. When a child is not learning in school, each of these factors must be evaluated and attempts made to modify the problems that are remediable. This is not a simple task.

Role of the neurologist

The role of the neurologist in the management of children with learning disabilities is to answer the questions that parents of these children ask: "What are we to do with our child to help him learn and behave?" "What are we to expect of him?" "Why does he have this problem?" Arriving at the answers to these questions is not only difficult, but also requires the skills and talents of professionals in several disciplines. The neurologist must be thorough in taking the history and performing the physical examination, not only to uncover clues to etiology and remediation, but also to impart to the parents the feeling that he is concerned about the problem, has investigated it thoroughly, and has some idea of how the learning problem has affected the family. This approach is necessary because the solution often involves a great deal of time and commitment of effort from both parents—a solution that will not be followed unless the family is convinced that the doctor, knowing their child well, has planned the best program of remediation.

Medical history

The medical history should begin with the recounting of the mother's pregnancy and labor, and the delivery of the child. Unless specific questions are asked about all details of the pregnancy and perinatal events, important clues may be overlooked. Parents, especially fathers, have a great propensity for forgetting details and answering the question "Were there any complications during pregnancy?" by merely saying, "No." Separate questions about maternal health, drugs, exposure to illness, spotting, weight gain, blood pressure, labor, delivery, condition at birth, etc. are answered more correctly. Information about prematurity, respiratory distress, jaundice, or other serious illnesses in the neonatal period should be specifically sought. Any serious illness in the child's life, particularly encephalitis or meningitis, can result in a significant central nervous system dysfunction that interferes with learning, and it will usually come to light if an inquiry is made about illnesses that have required hospitalization. Delayed developmental landmarks, especially in language function, indicate that the child is slow in maturation or is mentally retarded. Details about developmental milestones and academic records of relatives may indicate an inherited delay in central nervous system maturation by revealing problems in close relatives that are similar to the child's. The developmental history can be supplemented by reviewing the pediatrician's records or the child's baby book.

Evidence of any chronic illness that interferes with a child's attendance in school or lowers his stamina should be sought in the past history and review of systems. Questions regarding serious head trauma or seizure disorders are obviously important in obtaining clues about possible central nervous system damage or malfunction. Children, especially boys, with seizure disorders who are treated with phenobarbital sometimes become hyperactive and difficult to manage. Substitution of diphenylhydantoin (Dilantin) or primidone (Mysoline) for the phenobarbital may alleviate the child's behavioral problems.

Relationships between child and parents

Regardless of what other factors are operative in causing the child's learning disability, an understanding of how the child's behavior has affected the family is vital for dealing with the parents and planning a remedial program for the child. Each parent should be given an opportunity to respond to questions. Insight into the parents' feeling for the child is obtained by listening to their descriptive terms and watching their facial expressions as they answer questions and describe the child and his behavior. The behavioral history should begin with postpartum events. Maternal depression following delivery, family problems precipitated by the arrival of an unwanted infant, frequent crying without responsiveness to comforting, etc. complicate the early relationship between mother and child and may lead to maternal feelings of guilt and inadequacy, which in turn may lead to anger. These emotions must be recognized and their genesis discussed before they can be dealt with effectively. Discussing them openly with the physician in a neutral, understanding setting may be helpful.

The parents' ideas regarding the child's behavior should be explored to determine whether both recognize a behavioral problem, how they respond to it, and whether they have ideas regarding its genesis. One parent may feel that the child is being babied and that all he needs is discipline, whereas the other may feel that the demands made on the child are too great. If the parents do not agree about the cause or the existence of the child's problem, the difficulties involved in helping the child are considerably more complex and involve, among other things, the parents' reaching an agreement.

Specific forms of discipline should be discussed to determine the response of the child to physical punishment, banishment to his room, rewards for good behavior, etc. This information will suggest techniques that can be used to help the child in the learning situation. Inquiries about the difference in the length of a child's attention span when he is playing and when he is studying, about what he enjoys, and about what he particularly dislikes may give useful clues for planning a program of remediation. His performance in sports, his relationships with peers, and the ages of his playmates may suggest immature development socially and physically and should influence the therapeutic program that is developed.

The child's school performance and behavior are discussed with the parents. They should be asked about how he did in each grade, and which are his strong subjects and which are his weak ones. School reports may add important information and provide an opportunity to "check" the parents' story against the teacher's. Commonly, children with learning disabilities have been seen by other consultants before being referred to the neurologist, and their reports should be reviewed. Not only are the reports and suggestions of these consultants valuable, but the actions taken by the parents to put these suggestions into effect give additional information about the parents' cooperation and resoluteness.

A social history is important. Children with learning problems fairly commonly come from disrupted households. The child's behavior can be either a major cause of the parents' disagreement or a result of their disharmony. The stability of the family, major sources of disagreement, and the ability of the parents to discuss problems and reach compromise solutions are all factors that must be appreciated in planning a successful program to influence the child's behavior and learning.

In summary, the medical history outlined, with emphasis on perinatal, developmental, and especially behavioral aspects, is unusual in its attention to items generally considered "nonmedical." However, the information obtained is necessary for a complete understanding of the child's problems and must form the foundation of any remedial program.

NEUROLOGICAL EVALUATION

The physical examination may be entirely normal, since there are no physical findings diagnostic of learning disability. The general physical examination should include auditory and visual screening tests. Deviation from normal should result in further audiological or ophthamological evaluation. Evidence of any chronic illness should be sought, and for this reason plotting the child's growth on one of the standard growth grids is advisable. If the child's weight or height is significantly less than the third percentile, further medical evaluation may be indicated.

The most important aspect of the neurological examination is the mental status examination. Much of the necessary information can be ascertained by watching the child's behavior as the history is being obtained. How did he behave while the questioning was progressing? Did he play with one item or did he "get into everything"? If he misbehaved, what were his parents' reactions to his mischief? His speech and language should be noted and his intelligence estimated. The child's reading ability may be approximated by having him attempt to read a series of graded readers or paragraphs.

Obvious abnormalities, such as hemiplegia, increase the likelihood of structural damage in portions of the central nervous system that will impair learning. Additionally, and importantly, the child's self-concept and self-expectation are lowered by the physical effects of a significant neurological abnormality, further impairing his learning ability. Hyperventilation for 3 minutes, with careful observation for minor motor seizures, is rewarding on rare occasions. Such seizures may interfere with the child's ability to attend to the materials and lessons presented in the learning situation. Patterns of eye movements during reading are different in good readers from those in poor readers. The eyes of poor readers make more reversals when reading and are less able to keep on the line than those of good readers. This difference can as easily be the effect of poor reading as its cause, but it represents one of the only well-established physical difference between the groups. Impaired graphesthesia (ability to interpret letters or numbers traced on the skin), reported in some children with learning disabilities, is only another manifestation of their impaired reading ability, and not necessarily a sign of parietal lobe dysfunction.

"Minor," or "soft," neurological signs

A great deal of attention in the literature has been directed toward the neurological examination and the presence of "minor," or "soft," neurological signs in children with learning difficulties. Soft neurological signs refer to equivocal plantar reflexes (uncertain direction of movement of the large toe after stimulation of the sole of the foot), hyperactive deep tendon reflexes, unusually prominent saccadic (nonrhythmically jerky) eye movements noted on following, borderline choreoathetosis (characterized by involuntary writhing and jerky movements of the outstretched upper extremities), questionable ataxia or tremor on finger-to-nose testing, general awkwardness or clumsiness, prominent mirror movements of the upper extremities (when the child is performing a task with one arm, the other arm "mirrors" the movements), mild dystonias (abnormal, usually "stiff," postures of the extremities) that become evident when the child walks on his heels or the sides of his feet, or other equivocal findings for age. The difficulty of interpreting the significance of these signs, reflected in the adjectives "minor" and "soft," lies in the fact that these findings are *not definitely* abnormal as are other possible findings of a neurological examination, such as nystagmus (rhythmically jerky eye movements), but vary in amount with the age, maturity, intelligence, and cooperation of the child. The decision that they are abnormal in any child is a *subjective* decision, based partly on the other findings in the examination and largely on experience. These "abnormalities" appear in children without other evidence of neurological impairment and may be present on one examination and absent on later ones. The presence of soft neurological signs may be of importance in differentiating the child with learning problems from his normal classmates, but this is unlikely. Controlled studies are needed to determine the significance, if any, of these soft neurological signs, and even then it is likely that the presence of an equivocal plantar reflex, for example, will be only of statistical and not of therapeutic significance. The concept of "mixed cerebral dominance" is not sound. Cerebral dominance refers specifically and only to hemispheric control of language. The left cerebral hemisphere is "dominant" (in control of language) in right-handed as well as in most left-handed people. The existence, for example, of "right-eyedness" (with its bihemispheric connections), left-handedness, and right-footedness is undoubted but does *not* indicate mixed hemispheric control of language ("mixed cerebral dominance") but, rather, preferences that may not have a cerebral basis at all. Mixed eyedness, handedness, and footedness occur in learners as often as in nonlearners and, in any case, do not serve to explain the genesis of learning disabilities. The presence of right-left confusion in a child does not indicate cerebral damage but certainly will impair reading if the child cannot determine at which end of the word to begin reading. Therefore, an examination for the presence of right-left confusion should be performed.

The selection of laboratory tests that should be ordered depends on the information obtained during the history taking and physical examination as well as on the social and educational level of the parents and their consequent expectations. No "screening tests" are suggested.

Value of electroencephalography

A great deal of misdirected enthusiasm and mystical expectation has been directed toward electroencephalography in the management of children with learning disabilities. The popular thought is that an abnormal electroencephalogram (EEG) indicates abnormal brain function and that a normal EEG indicates that the brain is functioning normally. However, both assumptions are incorrect. There is no electroencephalographic abnormality diagnostic of learning disability. Excessive slow activity for age, a minor and nonspecific abnormality, is the most commonly reported "abnormality" seen in the EEG of children with learning problems and probably represents the electroencephalographic concomitant of central nervous system immaturity. Excessive slow activity may not be more common in these children than in normal ones. Children with histories suggestive of minor motor seizure disorders should have an EEG made. Those children with temper tantrums or paroxysmal abnormal behavior may also benefit if an EEG is obtained both while they are awake and while asleep.

If epileptogenic activity is seen, appropriate anticonvulsants may favorably alter their behavior and learning and are worth a trial. However, carefully controlled studies are necessary to establish the value of an EEG in planning the management of these children and of other children with learning problems, especially in view of the claims of improved learning and behavior in children receiving anticonvulsant medication, even in children without paroxysmal abnormal EEG's.

Parents often come to the neurologist expecting an EEG to be obtained, and that, perhaps, is the best indication for obtaining one. However, the high incidence of minor and nonspecific abnormalities present in EEG's of normal children and the inability of the physician to explain to the parents what a "minor EEG abnormality" indicates diagnostically, therapeutically, and prognostically make doubtful the value of obtaining routine EEG's of children with learning disabilities.

EVALUATION BY OTHER SPECIALISTS

After the medical and neurological evaluation has been completed (little, if any, of which requires the peculiar training and expertise of the neurologist), referral to other specialists is necessary. Severe emotional problems should be referred to a psychiatrist. If visual or auditory defects are detected, an ophthalmologist or audiologist should be consulted, and speech problems should be referred to a speech pathologist. Psychological consultation is nearly always indicated. Requests for an

"IQ test" are as useless to the psychologist as requests for an "EEG" are to the neurologist. The psychologist should be given background information about the child and his learning problem. The particular tests used for assessment of the child's intellectual ability, achievement levels, perceptual channels most open for learning, and personality are selected by the psychologist according to his professional training and experience. The information gained about the child's intellectual ability and achievement levels allows realistic goals to be established for the child. Additionally, thorough psycho-educational evaluation is important in establishing a base line so that the child's progress can be followed and the effect of the remedial program evaluated.

PROGRAM PLANNING FOR REMEDIATION

After the evaluation has been completed, the more difficult task is that of deciding on a program for remediation. The remedial program will vary according to the problems, strengths, and weaknesses of the child, his family situation, and the facilities available. The program must take these factors into account and should be jointly decided on in a meeting of the psychologist, a representative of the school, and the neurologist. The neurologist's or physician's role is important in this phase—not for making the decisions but for coordinating the professional people involved and relating the group's decisions, with explanations, to the family. It is quite likely that one of the other professionals could do as well or better in this phase, except that the physician, with his unique role in society, is especially suited to harmonize the group and to have the plan accepted by the parents. The plan should begin with a thorough discussion with the parents of the results of the evaluation and of the emotional impact of the child on the family and vice versa. Specific suggestions should be made to the parents about ways to alter favorably the emotional climate at home. Techniques of behavior modification should be described and a behavior modification program implemented. The child's school situation will require change or alteration, and finally consideration must be given to the use of psychoactive medications.

A summary of the evaluation should be presented to both parents, with an enumeration of possible causal factors if any have been uncovered. The detail or extent of this explanation will vary from family to family. If a cause for the child's learning problem has not been uncovered, this fact should be admitted; at the same time the parents should be reassured that no evidence of a brain tumor nor of progressive disease of the nervous system is present. It is surprising how often parents have these thoughts, especially if they have been told that their child "has something wrong with his brain" (minimal brain damage, minimal cerebral dysfunction, etc.). It is perhaps to these parents that the neurologist has the most to offer: the ability to reassure them that their child does not have an ominous disease of the brain. The doctor should acknowledge the frustration the parents experience because their child is not learning, and the parents should be subtly prompted to express their feelings of disappointment, anger, and resultant guilt. This discussion, with emphasis on how understandable and common these emotions are, can result in the lessening of parental guilt feelings and in a more reasonable and comfortable attitude toward their child. To help avoid further disappointments, the doctor should predict that the solution to the child's learning disability will be neither immediate nor easy. For that very reason, it may be wise to point out to the parents that their second grader has had seven years to develop his problem, and that it will not be solved immediately. Furthermore, if medications are used, it must be stressed that they are only a small part of the answer—not *the* answer.

Parental role

Parents need guidance in modifying emotions and conditions that interfere with their child's learning. Thus the results of the psychological reports should be discussed with them so that reasonable demands can be made on their child and so that realistic expectations can be formed; unrealistic expectations and demands cause continuing frustration and disappointment for both parents and child. The child is extremely sensitive to parental attitudes, and his reactions to their attitudes may further impair his ability to learn by lessening his expectations for success and by increasing his emotional difficulties. Specific suggestions should be made to the parents about handling their child. For example, children who are easily distracted from their studies should have a study area where disturbing stimuli can be limited. The parents should be told that children with learning disabilities require more firm and consistent discipline than their brothers and sisters. Attempts by the parents to divert their child's attention from some action that is annoying them to a different activity are much more effective than constantly having to reprimand him. The parents should be informed that the child's many disturbing, or "naughty," actions are often unintentional. This knowledge, coupled with advice to overlook many of these little offenses, will help prevent continuing confrontations between the child and his parents and thus ease tensions in the home. The parents can help restore a warm relationship with their child by talking to him in his room at bedtime after he has had time to settle down. Quiet conversation about the day's events, ended by verbalizing their love for him, can be very effective "therapy" for both parents and child.

BEHAVIOR MODIFICATION

Behavior modification should be used by the parents to increase the child's motivation to learn and to help alleviate behavior problems at home. Behavior modification is the term given to an approach to learning that was developed in the laboratory by experimental psychologists and that has proved to be successful when used with children. Perhaps because this method was developed by non-physicians and because of the parochial attitude of psysicians, it has not received the proper attention in the medical literature that it deserves. Briefly, behavior modification is a theory of learning that attributes the choice of action an organism makes when faced with a nonunique situation to the consequences or reinforcements which have followed that same choice on previous occasions. A child shows his "A" in spelling to his father, and the father tells him how proud he is. A good deal of the child's motivation to earn an "A" on the spelling test (the test being the nonunique situation) is his knowledge that his father will be quite proud of him when he brings the grade home. Pride expressed by the father to the child is the "reinforcement" or reward that helps perpetuate the child's good behavior. On the other hand, the child who slams the door each time he enters it, only to produce a minor tantrum in his mother, continues to slam the door because it elicits the response that he wants—some of his mother's attention.

Although the details of establishing a full program of behavior modification are out of the realm of the neurologist's competence and of this discussion, some of its components are straightforward enough that they can be taught to the parents and used to help the child with learning disabilities. The symptoms, or patterns of behavior, that are most disturbing to the parents are listed in a hierarchical order. For instance, if the child has no particular behavior pattern at home that is disturbing to his parents, then the first item on this list will be the child's learning problem in school. Next the situations that elicit or contribute to the unwanted behavior are noted. For example, it may be that the child's difficulties in school are due to his inability to concentrate while studying, or to an excessive amount of time wasted in watching television. Third, the factors that perpetuate the unwanted behavior, by acting as reinforcement to it, are considered. The parents' verbal and physical reactions to the child's failure must be analyzed as possible reinforcements to the child's unwanted behavior. Finally, a system of positive rewards for good performance and, much *less* important, of reasonable punishments for failure is worked out with the parents and the child. It is vital to stress to the parents that only one problem at a time be approached, that the demands for successful accomplishments be within the ability of the child, that all rewards and punishments immediately follow the good or bad behavior, and that the parents agree to the rewards as well as to the punishments. The early frustrations and the great amount of time required before significant changes will be seen must be stressed to the parents to help prevent their becoming disappointed and abandoning the program.

BEHAVIOR REINFORCEMENT

The rewards for good behavior need not be tangible objects. Expressions of pride, compliments, and praise are effective. Young children respond amazingly well to a "gold star" system whereby, for example, each time they do their spelling assignment they receive a gold star. For a child, the prospect of trading five or ten gold stars for a trip with his father can add further enticement to the system and provide motivation for good behavior. Attention to the child when he is good is one of the most effective reinforcements of good behavior that parents can use. A temptation that is understandable, but that worsens the situation with a difficult child, is to ignore him when he is good and to pay attention to him when he is bad by shouting or threatening punishment. This mistake is extremely common. The parents should be strongly encouraged to turn the situation around. When the child is good, the mother stops her household chores and reads to him, or the father puts his paper down and plays ball with him. This approach is difficult to carry out, since often the parents feel a sense of relief when the child is playing quietly and ignore him at this time. Substitution of good behavior for bad is another useful technique. It is much more effective to praise a child for working on his homework than to punish him for not completing it, and the parents should be encouraged to condemn less often and to offer more encouragement.

Negative reinforcement or punishment is also important in "extinguishing" bad behavior. Punishments should be considered beforehand so that useless threats are not made. Saying to the child, "If you don't turn off that TV, you can't go out for a month," is less effective than saying, "Turn off the TV or you can't go bowling on Saturday," because the latter can realistically be enforced. Sending a child to his room when he is misbehaving is effective if not overused. When the child's behavior requires punishment, he should be told, "Johnny, I love you, but I don't like you when you . . . ." This expression of love is extremely important to a child who is used to failure and to disappointing his parents, for it helps him maintain confidence in himself because it is reassuring to him. The verbalization of love for their child can also be important to the parents, as it may help them to renew some of their lost affection for this child who frequently disappoints them and disrupts their home.

Children with learning problems frequently look on themselves as being inferior to their classmates. Those with the additional handicap of being clumsy have an even more impaired self-image. Effective physical education directed at skills which the child must use on the playground with his peer group, or which allow him to compete successfully in one sport or another, will favorably alter the child's opinion of himself and of his time spent at school. No child enjoys being chosen last consistently during gym class. If his physical skills increase, the situation changes, and the child, instead of dreading the physical education program and consequently disliking school, will soon look forward to this time. The improved self-image that accompanies new physical abilities may well be the basis of the success claimed for the treatment of children with learning disabilities by certain physical education techniques, and makes at least as much sense as the concept of "enhancement of visual-motor perception through exercise."

School setting

Finally, the school setting may require change. Depending on the parents' financial situation, a private school, especially one oriented toward helping children with learning disabilities, may be of benefit to the child. The decision will depend on many factors, including the facilities available in the public school. Children with learning disabilities who attend Roman Catholic schools with large classrooms may do well to transfer to public schools if the classrooms are smaller, although in some instances the firmly structured setting of Roman Catholic schools may be beneficial. Changes are often difficult to accomplish in a school because of the provincialism of many school administrators and the lack of trained school personnel. Ideally, the school will have specialists in remedial education who will have the primary responsibility for the child's school program and who will have contributed their ideas and suggestions to the total therapeutic program. Where no specialists are present in the school system, a conference with the classroom teacher should be held and the results of the evaluation discussed. Suggestions are much more likely to be followed enthusiastically if the teacher has participated in the evaluation of the child and in the formulation of the remedial program. This makes her a partner in making the decisions and thus anxious to see that the program succeeds. Knowledge of the child's intellectual ability and achievement levels, as measured by the psychologist, is important so that realistic demands of the child can be made by the teacher. The achievement levels and whether the child learns best by the auditory, visual, or tactokinesthetic route must be known in order to plan an effective educational program. This is true whether the educational approach concentrates on the child's strengths or on his weaknesses. The actual educational techniques used by the teacher will depend on her background, experience, and resourcefulness, but the program should be tailored to the child rather than the reverse. For example, this approach may be especially helpful in establishing requirements for handwriting, as neatness may be beyond the child's physical ability. The lowering of standards for neatness may result in more acceptable performance and behavior from the child in other areas.

The techniques of behavior modification as outlined to the child's parents can be discussed with the teacher and applied in the classroom situation. The teacher, aware of the child's abilities and limitations, must provide opportunities for him to succeed and then must respond in a manner that reinforces this desired behavior. Subjects interesting to the child can be selected for his studies, and favorite activities can be used as rewards for good performance. It should be suggested to the teacher that the most effective technique in eliminating poor behavior in the classroom is to ignore the child when he misbehaves and to pay attention to him when he performs well.

Value of medication

Claims of dramatic improvement in behavior and learning subsequent to the initiation of medication are reported anecdotally in the literature and supported by remarkably few carefully controlled, double-blind studies. The criteria necessary to predict reasonably which child will benefit from medication and which will show no change or become worse are uncertain. It appears as though the hyperactive child with a medical history and neurological examination suggestive of central nervous system insult is more likely to respond favorably to medication than the child who is not hyperactive in the office, whose hyperactivity or misbehavior in the office is not challenged by his parents, who is bored in school because he is either too bright or too slow compared to his classmates, or who has emotional problems. Since no predictive criteria are established, it is reasonable to begin drug therapy on a trial-and-error basis. Methylphenidate (Ritalin), 10 mg., before breakfast and lunch, or dextroamphetamines in slightly smaller dosage are the drugs of choice; they have a paradoxical calming effect on some children with learning disabilities. Methylphenidate is given before meals to enhance its absorption. If no response is seen, the dosage can be increased gradually up to about 2 mg. per kilogram per day or until improvement or side effects are noted. Side effects with methylphenidate are unusual but may include a worsening of hyperactivity. With dextroamphetamines, the parents may complain of either a worsening of hyperactivity or of anorexia subsequent to the medication. These medications can be restricted to school days in an attempt to prevent the refractoriness that develops in some children with prolonged usage. If one drug does not work, the likelihood of the other being beneficial is lessened, but it may still be worth a trial. If neither is helpful, or if the child is made more hyperactive, diphenhydramine hydrochloride (Benadryl), thioridazine hydrochloride (Mellaril), or chlordiazepoxide (Librium) may be of benefit. A real concern about the possibility of drug abuse, either by other members of the family or by the child, exists. No one knows how a child who feels as though he "needs" medicine to be normal will react when he is older, and this concern should temper any decisions to continue prescribing medications for children who are receiving only questionable benefit from them.

The physician should schedule follow-up visits, frequently at first, and then less often, depending on the progress of the child. The major purpose of these follow-up visits is to discuss the results of the behavior modification program in order to determine whether the parents have initiated the suggestions made to them. If suggestions are made without a plan of continuing help, it is likely that the parents, after a feeble attempt at trying to initiate the suggestions, will forget them. Furthermore, the effect of follow-up visits is to use a technique of behavior modification on the parents, that is, to reinforce the parents' action of putting the plan into effect by expressing approval, or to use negative reinforcement by expressing disapproval if they have not done so. In addition, of course, the dosage and effects of medications are checked, and the child's behavior and school performance are followed.

In the future, attempts must be made to prevent learning disabilities and to improve our management of them. Improved prenatal care, more carefully monitored labor and delivery, better management of premature infants, removal of toxins from the environment, improved childhood nutrition, and less crowded schools are all important in the prevention of learning disabilities. Providing teachers who are well trained, enthusiastic, and capable of dealing with the different abilities of their students is of paramount importance and perhaps can be achieved by offering salaries commensurate with the vital role teachers have in influencing our children. Family physicians and pediatricians can help prevent learning problems. To do this, they must receive more training in the management of behavior problems, and they must devote more attention to the techniques of child rearing and to minor behavior problems during "well baby" and other office visits. Perhaps in the future, the nurse-practitioners will free the physician from his more routine chores so that the extra time required for attention to these matters will be available. Finally, carefully controlled studies designed to evaluate the effect of pharmacological agents and educational techniques on learning and behavior must be made. The identification of the characteristics of subgroups of children with learning disabilities who respond to one therapeutic approach better than another is vital so that remediation can be on a more rational basis.

SUMMARY

In summary, the term "learning disability" is defined. The frequency and causes of learning disabilities and the behavior characteristics of children with learning disabilities are discussed. A role is suggested for the neurologist or other physician in the evaluation and management of children with learning disabilities. The importance of a detailed behavioral history is stressed, and serious doubts are raised about the significance of "soft" neurological signs and of minor electroencephalographic abnormalities in the management of these children. The formulation of a remedial program is discussed and related to the data gathered during evaluation. In the program of remediation the vital importance of changing attitudes and of behavior modification at home and at school is emphasized, the use of medications is mentioned, and the value of follow-up visits is outlined. Finally, those areas deserving of more attention and research in order to prevent learning disabilities and to allow their management to be on a more rational basis are mentioned.

REFERENCES

Bettman, J. W., Stern, E. L., Whitsell, L. J., and Gofman, H. F.: Cerebral dominance in developmental dyslexia, Arch. Ophthal. **78:**722, 1967.
Conners, C. K., Eisenberg, L., and Barcai, A.: Effects of dextroamphetamine on children: studies on children with learning disabilities and school behavior problems, Arch. Gen. Psychiat. **17:**478, 1967.
Critchley, M.: Developmental dyslexia, Springfield, Ill., 1964, Charles C Thomas, Publisher.
Freeman, R. D.: Drug effects on learning in children: a selective review of the past thirty years, J. Spec. Ed. **1:**17, 1966.
Haring, N. G., and Lovitt, T. C.: Operant methodology and educational technology in special education. In Haring, N. G., and Schiefelbusch, R. L.: Methods in special education, New York, 1967, McGraw Hill Book Co.
Paine, R. S.: Syndromes of "minimal cerebral damage," Pediat. Clin. N. Amer. **15:**779, 1968.
Paine, R. S., and Clements, S. D.: Minimal brain dysfunction in children, Educational, Medical, and Health Related Services, N&SDCP monograph, publication no. 2015, Washington, D. C., 1969, United States Public Health Service.
Werry, J. S.: Developmental hyperactivity, Pediat. Clin. N. Amer. **15:**581, 1968.
Werry, J. S., and Wollersheim, J.: Behavior therapy with children: a broad overview, J. Amer. Acad. Child Psychiat. **6:**346, 1967.
Whitsell, L. J.: Learning disorders as a school health problem: neurological and psychiatric aspects, Calif. Med. **111:**433, 1969.
Yakovlev, P. I., and Lecours, A.: The myelogenetic cycles of regional maturation of the brain. In Minkowski, A., editor: Regional development of the brain in early life, Philadelphia, 1967, F. A. Davis Co.

chapter 9

USE OF DRUGS TO HELP CHILDREN WITH LEARNING PROBLEMS

MARK A. STEWART

The specific learning problems of children that we now recognize often seem to over-lap each other. Perhaps the reason is that such handicaps seldom come singly, but it could also be that we have not learned enough about the natural history of these conditions to put them together into syndromes. I am including the following difficulties under the general heading of problems that interfere with learning to read: (1) faulty development of visual perception, (2) faulty development of auditory perception, (3) poor coordination of fine and coarse movements, and poor articulation, (4) poor integration of visual perception and hand movements, (5) delayed development of the use or understanding of language, and (6) specific reading disability. This list does not imply that the specific problems occur on their own.

Genetic factors seem to operate in some of the conditions (for example, in delayed language development and reading disability), and brain damage can probably produce any or all of the difficulties, but it is fair to say that the origins of these problems are not yet understood. Sometimes the problems are accompanied by behavior such as overactivity and impulsiveness, an unhappy coincidence that seems most likely to follow a definite brain injury. Often a learning problem is compounded by the child's growing sense of defeat and waning self-confidence, and this complication becomes the most important factor in the overall prognosis.

PHYSICIAN'S ROLE

How can the physician help children with such problems, and when should he use drugs? I believe that drugs have only a small part in the management of learning problems, and that even this part will dwindle away as the schools become better equipped to work with children who have such handicaps. I would therefore like to review briefly the more important facets of the physician's role. In the first place the physician may be the one to organize the diagnosis. Because many schools do not yet have the personnel to evaluate children who are having difficulty in learning, parents turn to their family doctor or pediatrician for help. The physician can make a preliminary diagnosis of language disability or specific reading disability on the basis of a simple psychological examination consisting of a standard reading test (Gray Oral Reading Test), a screening test for intelligence (Raven's Coloured Progressive Matrices), a test of the child's ability to name common objects, and a spelling test. He would then refer the child to a competent clinical psychologist for a battery of tests that would define the specific blocks to learning and provide the basis for a teaching prescription. Some children will also need visual and auditory testing, as well as an examination of speech and language functions.

The physician is in a particularly good position to explain the results of the various tests to the parents and the child himself, to discuss the likely prognosis, and to pass on the analysis and suggested treatment to the child's teachers. Subsequently the responsibility for a direct attack on the learning problems rests with the teachers, speech therapists, and possibly physical therapists, but the physician still has a crucial role in helping the child to regain his self-confidence and his interest in learning. It is vital that he help the parents develop acceptance and understanding of the problem, advise them about effective ways to bolster the child's self-esteem, and persuade them not to try to teach the child themselves. The physician should reassure the child, pointing out that his difficulty in learning does not imply that he is dumb, nor that he will have as much trouble when he is grown up and at work as he is having in school.

EFFECTS OF STIMULANTS ON THE CHILD'S BEHAVIOR

Drugs play their part in the overall management by reducing some specific handicaps to learning and improving the child's attitude toward learning. In an ideal educational setting such artificial maneuvers would not be necessary, because a trained and interested teacher working with a small group of problem children excites her pupils to learn and can work around behavior such as restlessness and distractibility. However, in the real world, most children with learning problems are taught in classrooms where the teachers have neither the skill nor the time to cope with behavior that prevents a child from finishing his work and that may disrupt the class. In an ordinary classroom the child with problems feels inferior to his peers and senses the teacher's frustration. A vicious circle starts in which the original difficulty is compounded by the child's embarrassment and discouragement, which in turn leads to his ceasing to try, and to further frustration for the teacher. Drugs can be a first-aid treatment for the child's morale by improving his learning habits, getting him back into the class routine, and persuading him that he has the ability to succeed.

What drugs can be used, and what functions will they affect? The stimulants amphetamine and methylphenidate seem to be by far the most useful. Experimental studies have shown that these drugs have a variety of effects on the performance of normal subjects, some of which have an obvious relationship to the effects of drugs on learning problems. It is well established, for example, that amphetamines lengthen the time during which a normal subject will perform a dull monitoring task at an optimal level; in other words, the drug seems to improve the ability of people to concentrate on, and persevere with, a boring task. It is also established that amphetamines produce feelings of well-being and confidence, and outgoing behavior. Stimulants may also improve coordination. These effects on normal subjects seem rather similar to the stimulants' action of lengthening the concentration of distractible children, improving the general attitude of children with learning problems, and occasionally producing better handwriting and tidier work. On the other hand, the calming effect of stimulant drugs on children with behavior problems, the diminishing of restlessness, and the apparent alleviation of impulsiveness seem to be exactly the opposite of effects noted in normal subjects.

Carefully controlled studies have produced some evidence that stimulant drugs improve the performance of children with learning problems on tasks resembling the regular assignments of school. However, the experimental demonstrations of improved performance come nowhere near matching the teachers' and parents' reports of striking improvement in the children's general behavior, performance, and attitudes. It seems clear that the stimulant drugs produce an improvement in many difficult children in the eyes of the teachers and parents, but we cannot be sure that there are specific effects on the children's actual learning. A shortcoming of the studies in this field is that the children studied have been diagnosed only in a general way as having learning or behavior difficulties; there is therefore no information on whether the drugs affect specific learning problems. Until the necessary studies are made it seems reasonable to try giving drugs to any child with a learning problem, particularly when the child's learning is complicated by a short attention span or a behavior problem such as restlessness and impulsiveness.

Dosage regulation

How should such drugs be given? It is important, first, to explain to the parents why the drugs are being prescribed and to reassure them that the use of stimulant drugs for their child's problem is an accepted part of medical practice. Second, one must be specific about the timing of medication. Drugs should be prescribed so that they will cover the child through his day in school and no more. The long-term benefits to children with learning and behavior problems are the result of the drug's restoring their confidence in their ability to do schoolwork rather than controlling their behavior throughout the day.

Children who improve while receiving stimulant drugs usually derive the most benefit from dextroamphetamine (Dexedrine), 5 mg., or methylphenidate (Ritalin), 10 mg. The action of these dosages, given in tablet form, lasts from 4 to 6 hours, and the school day can therefore be conveniently covered by giving a dose at breakfast and a dose at lunch. It is wise to start children at a lower dosage level, since a higher level may affect a child in the opposite direction, thereby scaring the parents and perhaps permanently discouraging them from using this kind of treatment. A cautious approach is to prescribe 5 mg. of Ritalin (or its equivalent,

2.5 mg. of Dexedrine) in a single dose to be given at breakfast time for one week. The dosage can then be raised to 10 mg. twice a day in steps if there is no effect or only a slight one. While some clinicians advise giving children 30 mg. or more of Dexedrine a day, I believe the side effects of such dosages are likely to outweigh the benefits. Even at the dosage I suggest as a routine, some children will lose their appetite, have obvious letdowns, with worsening of behavior in the evening, and experience symptoms of anxiety such as nausea, stomachaches, irritability, and nervousness. As the dosage is increased from the level of 10 mg. of Ritalin twice a day, the incidence of side effects rises sharply, and beyond the level of 40 mg. of Ritalin a day, or 20 mg. of Dexedrine a day, there is a definite risk that a child will fall into a zombielike state in which he is crying continually, moves around very little, and has frightening illusions or hallucinations. Furthermore, there are very few children who benefit from high dosages of stimulants but not from more modest amounts.

Children are sensitive about taking drugs of this kind, fearing that their friends will consider them "crazy" or retarded if they find out about them. On the other hand, children cannot be trusted to take the lunchtime dose on their own. It is therefore best that the parents leave a supply of the pills with the school nurse or the principal's secretary and that the school arrange for the child to take the second pill of the day privately under the supervision of this person. Teachers should not be asked to administer the pill in the classroom, and they should be advised never to mention the subject in public. Unfortunately some teachers will make remarks in front of the class that tell everything: "You haven't taken your pill today Johnny; I can see it." One solution to the problem of giving the second pill at school is to give a child his Dexedrine in a Spansule form at the beginning of the day. The drawback to this method is that the absorption from Spansules is unpredictable; it is not uncommon for a child taking a 5 mg. Spansule at breakfast to have enough of the drug left in him at bedtime so that he has difficulty going to sleep.

Children seldom seem to develop tolerance to Dexedrine when it is given in the way described here—that is, only on school days. Tolerance to Ritalin is quite common after one or two months on the drug, but it is usually possible to compensate for this by increasing the dosage. Alternatively, one can simply switch to the equivalent dosage of Dexedrine. In rare cases, when tolerance to both drugs develops, one can switch at intervals from one drug to the other.

The specter of children abusing such drugs is a real one. Some enterprising grade-school children will try more of their pills with the idea of becoming even smarter, if the supply is in their hands. Dramatic anxiety and hyperventilation attacks may follow this overdosage. Fortunately most children of this age despise taking the pills and are not introspective enough to realize the effects of the drugs on their performance and attitudes to school work. This happy state of affairs stops when children reach junior high school. Some may then start selling pills to their friends or using the drugs to manipulate their mood. As far as I know there have been no studies on the question of whether children who have received drugs in grade school are more likely to abuse them later. This serious question needs to be answered. For the moment one has to weigh the advantages to a young child of taking the drug against the possible disadvantages later in life. Children with serious behavior or learning problems often grow so discouraged and resentful in their grade-school career that they become dropouts and delinquents, chronically at odds with society. The advantages of giving the drug may therefore outweigh the possible disadvantages considerably. On the other hand, it seems foolhardy to give stimulant drugs to children who have grown beyond the grade-school age. Teen-age children who need such treatment should probably receive imipramine hydrochloride (Tofranil) or amitriptyline (Elavil), drugs that are less likely to be abused. There is preliminary evidence that these drugs have the same effects on children as stimulants, but they should not be substituted for the familiar stimulants in younger children since their actions are more complicated, lasting, and potentially dangerous. The Federal Drug Administration has not approved an indication for the use of these drugs in children under the age of 12 years, so that a physician prescribing them for younger children should be careful to obtain "informed consent" from the parents.

OTHER REDUCTIONS

Many other drugs have been used to try to help children with learning or behavior problems: anticonvulsants, phenothiazines, and a variety of drugs with mixed tranquilizing and stimulant effects. Phenothiazines are quite often used to calm the driven behavior of the brain-damaged child, a favored drug being thioridazine hydrochloride (Mellaril). Phenothiazines will slow down such children, but their effect is usually transitory as tolerance develops quickly. These drugs have the major disadvantage for children with learning problems of reducing school performance and slowing mental processes. Diphenylhydantoin (Dilantin) has been given to children with behavior problems, but there is no evidence that this toxic drug improves behavior or learning.

EFFECTS OF DRUG USE

Finally something needs to be said about how one can find out whether a drug is helping a child in school. The relaying of the teacher's comments by parents to the physician is unsatisfactory. One can obtain a better idea of how a child is doing by directly communicating with the teacher, and such communication serves a number of other useful purposes. Teachers often misunderstand the use of drugs in children with problems and are prejudiced against this kind of treatment, just as parents may be. Unless this misunderstanding is cleared up, a teacher's reports may be highly colored by her disapproval of the drugs. By calling the teacher, one can also obtain the best information about side effects and learn most quickly about the development of tolerance. Direct communication with the teacher also allows the physician to pass on the psychologist's advice about specific teaching methods, or the comments of a speech therapist and other consultants, and to have an immediate feedback about the child's general psychological state as well as his progress in learning.

REFERENCES

Conners, C. K., and Eisenberg, L.: The effects of methylphenidate on symptomatology and learning in disturbed children, Amer. J. Psychiat. 120:458, 1963.

Conners, C. K., Eisenberg, L., and Barcai, A.: Effect of dextroamphetamine on children, Arch. Gen. Psychiat. 17:478, 1967.

Conners, C. K., Rothschild, G., Eisenberg, L., Schwartz, L. S., and Robinson, E.: Dextroamphetamine sulfate in children with learning disorders, Arch. Gen. Psychiat. 21:182, 1969.

Francis-Williams, J.: Children with specific learning difficulties, Oxford, 1970, Pergamon Press.

Smith, G. M., Weitzner, M. Levenson, S. R., and Beecher, H. K.: Effects of amphetamine and secobarbital on coding and mathematical performance, J. Pharmacol. Exp. Ther. 139:100, 1963.

Weiss, B., and Laties, V. G.: Enhancement of human performance by caffeine and the amphetamines, Pharmacol. Rev. 14:1, 1962.

Weiss, G., Werry, J., Minde, K., Douglas, V., and Sykes, D.: Studies on the hyperactive child. V. The effects of dextroamphetamine and chlorpromazine on behavior and intellectual functioning, J. Child Psychol. Psychiat. 9:145, 1968.

INDEX